Table of content

Introduction..

What is Insulin? 7

Be Very Veggie 11

Avoid Artificial Sweeteners 12

Beat the Diabetes 13

What is the Glycemic Index? 14

Super Foods 15

Diet Plan for Preventing, Controlling, and Curing Diabetes 20

Garlic Shrimp Linguine 22

Pot Roast Soup 24

Curry-Lime Chicken with Salad 26

Baked Butternut Squash 29

Baked Chicken Tenders 31

Panko and Parmesan Topped Zucchini 33

Veggie Burritos 35

Beef and Zucchini Meatballs 37

Roasted Chickpeas 39

Meatballs with Spaghetti	41
Lasagna Rolls	43
Lentil Soup	45
Irish Beef Pot Pie	47
Vanilla French Toast	49
Reuben Sandwich	51
Mashed Potatoes	53
Lemon Herb Pot Roast	55
Lima Beans	57
Oats and Quinoa Breakfast	59
Avocado Toast	61
Bean Soup with Kale	63
Stir-fried Chicken	65
Cheesy Quesadillas	67
Cucumber Salad	69
Beef Macaroni	71
Roasted Briskets	73
Veggie Stuffed Pita	75
One-Pot Paella	77

Comfort Shepherd's Pie 79

Lo Mein Noodles 82

Chicken and Dumplings Soup 84

Sugar-free Pumpkin Bread 86

Chickpea Flour Tortilla 88

Applesauce Brownies 90

No-Bake Strawberry Cheesecake 92

Sugar-free Blueberries Coffee Cake 94

Berry Green Smoothie 96

Fruits Salad 98

Pineapple Salsa 100

Strawberries Salad 102

Creamy Lime Pie 104

Soda Pop Cake 106

Caramel Corn Crunch 108

Sugar-free Cookies 110

Sugar-free Frosting 112

Strawberry and Orange Drink 114

Sugar-free Pina Colada 116

Spinach and Artichoke Dip 118

Springtime Dip 120

Spicy Red Sauce 122

Introduction

Prediabetes and type 2 diabetes cases are increasing day by day around the world. An inactive and stressed lifestyle has increased the diagnosed cases of diabetes in individuals. Like many others, you might also assume that your life is already over when you are diagnosed with diabetes.

The meals and lifestyle change suddenly, and you get to know that now you have to think twice or more before eating anything available. This way, you cannot help yourself but getting panic. The doctor's advice and descriptions of blood sugar level and insulin become an announcement of your life pleasures getting over – forever. You find yourself being on a diet for the rest of your life, and it can be quite shutting down for you. But wait, although it is all true, things can be different.

Diagnosing diabetes is not the end of your life. You can still enjoy it; you can eat even many of your favorite foods. Basically, you can have it all, and you just need to be smart enough to manage things and make them appropriate accordingly. This diabetic diet cookbook is designed for everyone out there. It is for:

- All people who have diabetes to help them cope with specific events while taking perfectly good care of themselves in maintaining their blood sugar level.
- All those who care about someone who has diabetes.
- All the family members who want to include the diabetic loved ones in their celebrations.

This cookbook is specially designed in order to give you the tools that you might need for managing your insulin resistance while keep continuing to eat the food you want.

The most important thing you should keep in mind is that your major goal for diabetes management is learning how you can balance your blood sugar level by your physical activities as well as food. You should learn how different foods affect the blood sugar level of your body.

It is a lifetime methodology, not a seasonal plan. If you will follow the proper tools and manage things like a pro, you will notice positive changes in yourself in a few weeks. But another important thing is that do not stop the diet even if you reach the goal. It is not hard to learn, and it will also make you look great and feel perfect.

The Blood Sugar Briefing

When we go deep down for blood sugar, we actually mean blood glucose, which is a measure of glucose or sugar in your blood at any given time. When you eat something, your body digests it and breaks it into three macronutrients; carbohydrates, fats, and proteins.

Carbohydrates are further broken down in simple glucose that is absorbed in the bloodstream. That glucose then is transported in your body for your organs to get energy. Most of the glucose is used immediately, while others get stored for later use.

What is Insulin?

Insulin is one of the hormones. This organ releases insulin, which opens the cell doors and takes the sugar from the blood. Sugar is converted into energy when it enters the cells.

This keeps one keep going in their daily work. On the contrary, if the sugar does not get into the cells, you can feel anxious, shaky, mentally upset, and sweaty. It means the sugar in blood increases, and you develop insulin resistance. In this condition, the body does not use insulin properly, and the body needs more insulin for lowering the blood sugar level.

Prediabetes

The prediabetes is a condition in which a person's blood sugar level is higher than normal but not too high. The persons suffering from prediabetes are more vulnerable to get to type 2 diabetes, but there are researches that show that if you are a prediabetes patient, you can lower down the risk of next level diabetes by 58 percent, which seems to be quite promising. You can take precautions and follow proper meal plans with physical activities to knock it down.

Type 2 Diabetes

If you get detected with type 2 diabetes, then it clearly shows that your body is facing quite much insulin resistance. If your blood sugar level increases, it can cause some serious complications like nerve damage, heart, or kidney failures.

Risk Factors

With overweight or being 45 or above, there are many other risk factors involved in prediabetes and diabetes. They may include being physically inactive, having a parent or sibling with diabetes, or having high blood pressure.

Change Your Recipes

The basic thing is to take the food that goes with your body, not against it. You can have everything you want like mac n cheese, mashed potatoes, or stir-fried chicken, but with little transformations, you can make them your body friendly. The proper eating can actually reverse the insulin resistance and lower your risk for the disease. Keep following proper things to make any dish.

Go-To Grains

In the grains, always choose whole grain options. For making baked items like muffins or pieces of bread, use the whole wheat flour or oat bran in place of white flour. For pasta, also choose whole wheat pasta or sprouted grain. Whole wheat contains more fiber per serving. Also, prefer less processed food and also choose the ingredients with sugar in its third or beyond ingredient.

Natural fibers are less processed in any food, so prefer the food with more fiber. Also, pieces of bread, cookies, and other foods like this are typically not rich with fiber until unless fiber is add in them while processing. So, eating that food in a large quantity is not recommended. That is why find out the products made of sprout wheat or cereal with millet and flax that are not refined to add in fiber.

Talking about Bread

You should not eat bread that is too high in fiber or too low in carbs. Keep things moderate to enjoy healthy food. Try to replace white flour with whole wheat, spelled flour, oat bran flour, or sprouted flour in the slices of bread. Make sure to stick with unprocessed food as much as possible for you. There are many whole grain wheat products available to choose from as great options.

Balanced Diet with Beans

Beans are a superfood. They have proteins and carbohydrates and also packed with vitamins, fiber, and they can lower the cholesterol level. Beans are not only diabetes-friendly but heart-friendly too. You can buy the dry and overnight soaked beans as well as the canned ones. Just read the ingredients and nutritional facts to make sure that there is no added sugar in the canned items.

Dairy Facts

For balancing the blood sugar level in your body, keep in mind a few things like choose 1 percent milk only if you are using cow's milk. Almond, sunflower and soy milk should be unsweetened and fortified with vitamin and calcium. If you are using almond milk, make sure it is full of protein.

Flavor Yourself with Fruits

Fruits fall in carbohydrates family, and they can be great for us, but it is good to eat in moderate quantities. It is better to eat them mixed with other foods. Go for two servings of fruits per day. It is found out that ripe fruits are more likely to increase the sugar in your blood as when the fruit ripens, the complex sugars break down and raise the blood sugar level. So, it is good to go for less-ripe fruits as they remain in their complex form and do not break down quickly. Five fruits that contain 15 grams of carbs are 1 small apple (4 ounces), 1 small banana (4 ounces), ¾ cup berries, 17 small grapes (3 ounces), and 1 small orange (6.5 ounces).

Be Very Veggie

Vegetables are the rich source of carbs, and they can be eaten in quantity and variety. Basically, there are two types of vegetables, starchy and non-starchy. The root of the plant comes under the category of starchy vegetables like potatoes, sweet potatoes, beets, radish, jicama, and turnip.

Other such vegetables are butternut squash, pumpkin, corn, peas, and zucchini. On the other hand, non-starchy vegetables are cruciferous veggies like kale, spinach, chard, cauliflower, and broccoli.

You have to use many vegetables to affect your blood sugar level like three cups of raw non-starchy or 1 ½ cup of cooked non-starchy vegetables are equal to 15 grams. At least eat three servings of vegetables on a daily basis so go ahead and eat to your full and make your meal bowls colorful.

Avoid Artificial Sweeteners

Since people have been cutting out sugar from their diets by thinking that they can reduce the effects of real sugar, they have been moving to artificial sweeteners like Equal, NutraSweet, Sweet'N Low, SugarTwin, and Splenda. But no matter how much these little packs of sweeteners seem harmless, these are chemicals. Although they don't affect the glycemic response, they increase the cravings for sweet food items, and they also carry high calories.

There are some common natural sweeteners that can satisfy your sweet tooth. The following serving sizes of them are equivalent to 1 cup of white sugar:

- 1 teaspoon pure Stevia
- 2/3 cup agave nectar
- ¾ cup honey
- ¾ cup maple syrup
- 1 cup brown sugar

What is Stevia?

Stevia is a natural sugar that is found in the leaves of a plant named as Stevia. This natural sugar is 200 times sweeter than regular white sugar, and it also does not affect the blood sugar level in the body. It is a real sugar alternative but makes sure to buy 100 percent original one.

Mix Up the Meals

When you are going to eat, make sure you have a balanced diet. A balance of carbs (high in fiber foods should be preferred), proteins, and healthy fats like nut butter, canola oil, walnuts, salmon, and flaxseeds. For better lifestyles, eat these foods together. It is because the protein and fats in the food slow down the absorption of sugar in the blood. So, eating mixed food with fats, proteins, and carbs is the ideal and best way to manage your blood sugar, insulin resistance, and diabetes.

Beat the Diabetes

For beating down diabetes, you need to manage the foods that may are sugary and starchy and contain carbs. It really does not mean that cutting off the carbs from your diet is the answer. No, it is not. Rather some steps can be taken to balance out the blood sugar level by eating foods by combining with other foods for lowering the level of blood glucose in your body.

What is the Glycemic Index?

It is better to regularly get your blood glucose level either at home or through your doctor. Through this, you can easily identify what foods are leading your blood sugar to a higher level. It has the benefit that you can know which food is harmful to you and which foods you can keep continuing with.

Foods that have more effect on your blood sugar level are the ones with a higher glycemic index known as GI. It is an indicator of how fast a portion of food has the ability to raise your blood sugar level. Every food has a GI ranking and here is a list that shows the food with high or low GI.

High GI food includes white rice, white bread, and food made with white bread, breakfast cereal like cornflakes, cheerios, etc., potatoes and food made of them like French fries, potato dips, etc., sugary foods like cookies, cakes, candies, and donuts. The low GI foods are fruits and vegetables, wholemeal bread, wholemeal pasta, porridge oats, and lentils.

If you will eat the foods with high GI occasionally, it is not much risk to cause any diabetic problem in the long run, but if you consume these things on a regular basis, it may lead you to type 2 diabetes. It is better to combine high and low GI foods to balance out the risk.

Super Foods

Superfoods are a term that is used for describing a portion of food, which is particularly nutritious and high in health boosters like vitamins and minerals. Most of the vegetables and fruits are superfoods, and most of them are also with a low GI, so that is why they are great for diabetes. Some of them are:

Almonds – Almonds are found to be higher in fiber, and it helps to slow down the digestion process. They are also high in healthy fats and proteins, so they are perfect for portion control as a small amount of them can work for making you feel satisfied and fuller for a long time. Almonds are the food with relatively low GI. Adding them to your diet can lower down the risk of diabetes.

Apples – they are one of the richest sources of antioxidants. They are also low GI food and full of Vitamin C. Antioxidants are those minerals and vitamins that help to protect a body from high damaging effects of free radicals that are the chemicals that your body produces for its natural defense against the bacteria. Vitamin C boosts up the immune system of your body in a healthy way.

Bananas – They are also packed with antioxidants like apples. With that, they have the special property that they are a rich source of getting potassium in your body, which helps in blood pressure.

Beans – beans beings, a rich source of antioxidants, also are perfect for giving your body proteins and fiber. In fact, red beans, black beans, and kidney beans are the richest source beta-glucans, which helps to slow down the digestion of carbs and reduces the effect on blood sugar after eating.

Blueberries – the blueberries are packed with antioxidants, and their consumption can be quite helpful in lowering the blood sugar levels. Frozen berries are also as healthy as fresh ones.

Coconut and Coconut Oil – the coconut and coconut oil carries the properties that can reverse your diabetes. Research shows that if you use three to four tablespoons of coconut over your meals or snacks, you can get some amazing health improvements for diabetes of both types.

Ginger – Ginger is a source of anti-inflammation. It helps in dropping down the blood sugar levels.

Green Leafy Vegetables – Green leafy vegetables should be an essential part of your diabetic diet. They are all rich in health-boosting antioxidants. Broccoli is believed to be having an antioxidant that is actually helpful in reversing the artery damage caused by high blood sugar. Spinach also combats diabetes in a powerful and amazing way that you can imagine.

Cabbage – Cabbage is a source of vitamin C, vitamin K, and vitamin E. This is also full of beta carotene and potassium. Vitamin K is known for forming many proteins in the body.

Broccoli – a big and rich source of vitamin C, broccoli is perfect for fighting with high blood sugar. It also contains iron, beta carotene, and potassium, as well as high in bioflavonoids and antioxidants.

Spinach – Spinach is full of carotenoids that includes lutein and beta carotene. They are powerful antioxidants, and they also contain potassium and vitamin C.

Kale – a good source of calcium, beta carotene, iron, and vitamin C, kale is an amazing superfood.

Collard Greens – they are the source of omega 3 fatty acids that have anti-inflammatory properties.

Parsley – the one cup of parsley has 2 grams of proteins, and it is also full of calcium. They provide copper, iron, potassium, zinc, magnesium, beta carotene, vitamin C, and phosphorus.

Watercress – it contains vitamin C, iron, and beta carotene. It has 91 percent of water, which is also very useful for boosting up the hydration level in the body.

Sorrel – Sorrel is full of magnesium, calcium, and iron.

Dill – They contain iron, vitamin C, manganese, beta carotene, and calcium.

Basil – Basil provides your body with iron, manganese, copper, potassium, and beta carotene.

Coriander – coriander offers a peppery and mild flavor and also carries anti-inflammatory properties. They are full of vitamin C, magnesium, and iron.

Green vegetables and fruits contain chlorophyll that stimulates the production of hemoglobin and the oxygen-carrying pigments in red blood cells.

Green Tea – green tea is helpful in preventing the onset of type 2 diabetes. It is high in antioxidants and catechins that also provide great protection against diseases like cancer.

Honey – using natural honey can lower the blood glucose level when you use it as a sugar substitute. It also comprises of many other minerals and vitamins that can boost up the health.

Nuts – Nuts have the ability to provide the body with proteins and fat if you eat them in moderate quantity. Those who eat a handful of nuts everyday carry the 27 percent lower risk of type 2 diabetes development than those who do not eat them. The top nuts that can be eaten for diabetes are almonds, cashews, pecans, walnuts, pistachios, and other nuts from a tree nut.

Oily Fish – The omega 3 essential fatty acid content in the oily fish like salmon, sardines, trout, and mackerel are the perfect and healthy addition to any kind of diet. The human body is capable enough to make its own supply of fats as it stores excess protein and carbs coming from the food you consume, but there are some certain essential unsaturated fats, and the body gains them directly from the food you eat.

These essential oils are omega 6 and omega 3, and they come from oily fish, green leafy vegetables, and a few vegetable oils. Omega 3 reduces the inflammation in the body and reduces the risk of developing heart disease as well as other diseases like asthma and depression. On the other hand, omega 6 oils also carry some great health benefits, but they need to be consumed in a specific quantity; otherwise, they can lead to inflammation in your body. So, it is better to balance the consumption of omega 3 and omega 6 fatty oils.

White Vinegar – both white and red wine vinegar helps to lower down the blood glucose level in the body. If you do not use vinegar, then using lemon juice can work as it can give you the same positive impacts.

Yogurt – yogurt is a healthy and rich source of protein, and it also helps in reducing the blood sugar level in the body. Yogurt also cuts the belly fat when eaten as a part of a calorie control diet. But keep in concentration that not all yogurts are the same. Some brands use large quantities of sugar while processing, which is not good for diabetes. So it is better to choose plain yogurt from organic brands. If you want to add the sweetness, then add fresh fruits or honey in it according to your taste.

Diet Plan for Preventing, Controlling, and Curing Diabetes

For preventing, controlling, and curing diabetes, you can follow this diet plan having three steps:

Step 1 – Lower the Blood Sugar Level

You should try to lower down the blood sugar level in this step, and for this, you need to cut the carbs from your diet. You may have to skip some favorite foods of yours, but it is worth not to eat them. Food that you need to cut from your diet are some fats and starchy carbs containing food like wheat products, bread crumbs, pretzels, potatoes, chips, barley, vegetable oil, dairy products, corn, popcorn, beans, peas, soups, tortilla, and fruits like apples, oranges, papaya, cherries, pears, grapes, etc. You need to cut off soda, even diet soda from your diet as it can increase the risk of diabetes development in the individuals.

Step 2 – Eat for good health

In this step, you need to introduce healthy carbs in your diet, and you can also increase the consumption from 20 grams to 40 grams per day. But your aim should be to maintain the blood sugar level to 100 or lower to 80. In step 1, you cut many carbs from your diet, but in this step, you can bring them back. You can eat fruits and vegetables, low-fat dairy, and whole grains.

In this step, you will learn how some certain food affects your body after consumption. It is a critical phase, and you gradually assess your health and blood glucose levels. If you feel bloated or tired after eating some certain food, it is not a good choice.

Step 3 – Maintain Healthy Blood Sugar Level

In this step, you will start eating healthy for the rest of your life. A diabetic plan is not about just eating for a phase, but it is for a lifetime. In this phase, you will reduce the medications and maintain the blood sugar level by consuming healthy food. In the first two steps, you will see that it is true that you are what you eat. By cutting down the carbs and then introducing them again gradually, you can make some connection in the food you eat and how you feel after eating them.

In a regular diet, you need to eat the food that helps your body with preventing, controlling, and curing diabetes.

Garlic Shrimp Linguine

"Enjoy this amazing and yummy garlic shrimp linguine with your desired noodles. They are diabetic friendly and a perfect meal."

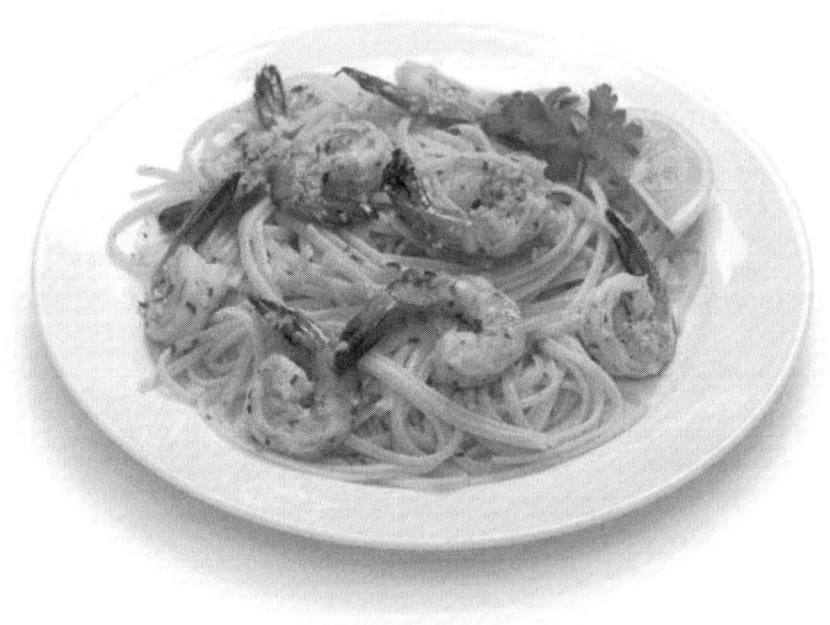

Prep Time:	10 minutes	Calories:	270
Cook Time:	15 minutes	Fat (g):	7g
Total Time:	25 minutes	Protein (g):	21g
Servings:	4	Net carbs:	30g

Ingredients:

- Uncooked multigrain linguine   6 ounces
- Raw shrimp, peeled and deveined   ½ pound
- Grated parmesan cheese   ¼ cup
- Diet margarine   3 tbsp
- Garlic clove, minced   One
- Seafood seasoning   ½ tsp
- Chopped parsley, optional   ¼ cup
- Salt, optional   1/8 tsp

Instructions:

1. Cook the linguine following the instructions.
2. Add in shrimp and cook for almost 5 minutes and then drain.
3. Now add in cheese, garlic, seasoning, margarine, and mix well to coat.
4. Now add in salt and parsley if using. Mix and serve.

Pot Roast Soup

"Make this amazing recipe of roast soup in your kitchen and enjoy a healthy diet."

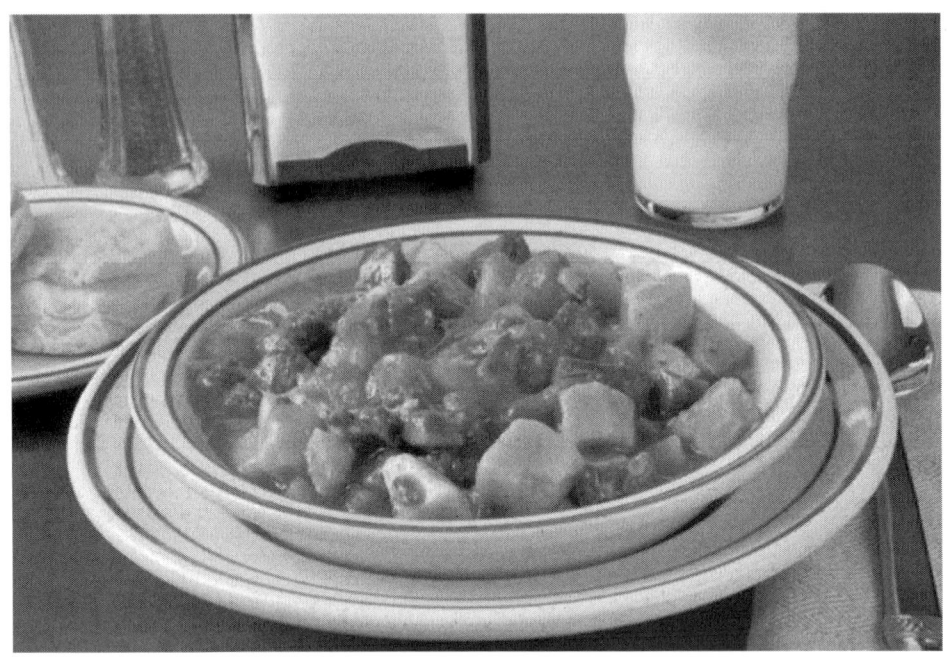

Prep Time:	10 minutes	Calories:	295
Cook Time:	7 hours	Fat (g):	8g
Total Time:	7 hours 10 minutes	Protein (g):	35g
Servings:	6	Net carbs:	17g

Ingredients:

- Beef shoulder roast boneless — 2 ½ pounds
- Onions, chopped — 2 cups
- Diced tomatoes — 15 ounces
- Hash brown potatoes, cubed — 1 cup
- Beef broth — 1 cup
- Minced garlic — 1 tbsp
- Dried thyme leaves — 1 tsp
- Pepper — ¼ tsp
- Broccoli slaw — 2 cups
- Frozen peas — ½ cup

Instructions:

1. Cut roast in equal pieces.
2. Place in a slow cooker and add in onions, tomatoes, broth, thyme, garlic, and pepper.
3. Cover and cook for 5 to 6 hours on high until beef is tender.
4. Add in broccoli and cook for half an hour.
5. Add in peas and cook more.
6. Serve after done.

Curry-Lime Chicken with Salad

"Make this exciting recipe for enjoying lunch or dinner. It is a simple diet for diabetic patients and a great source of fiber."

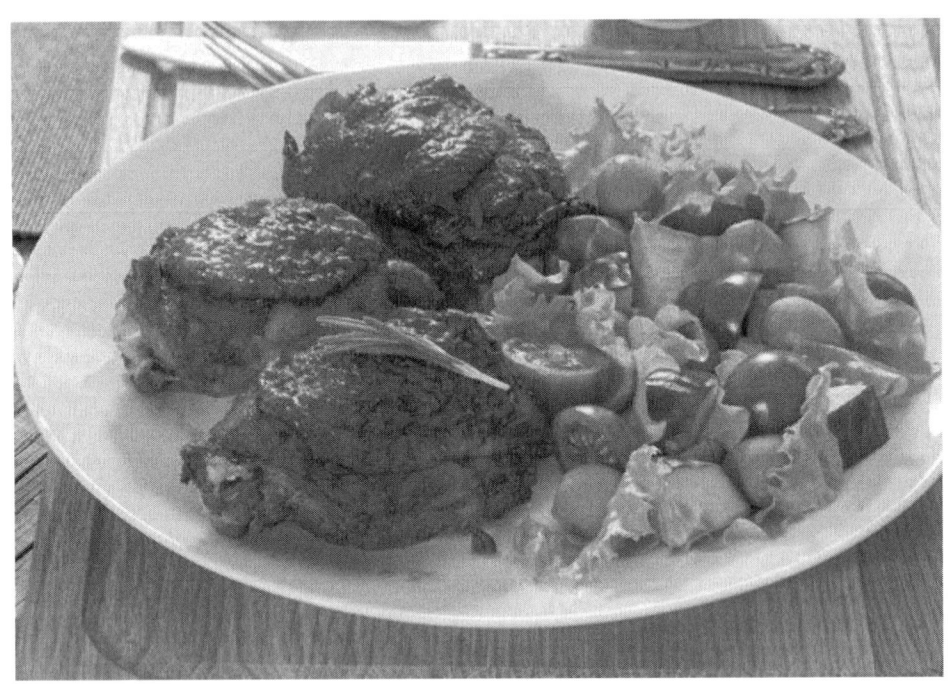

Prep Time:	1 hour 10 minutes	**Calories:**	400
Cook Time:	1 hour 20 minutes	**Fat (g):**	19g
Total Time:	2 hours 30 minutes	**Protein (g):**	33g
Servings:	4	**Net carbs:**	20g

Ingredients:

- Chicken thighs — 2 pounds
- Greek yogurt — 1 cup
- Diced ginger — 1 tsp
- Curry powder — 1 tsp
- Lime juice — One lime
- Red cider vinegar — 1 cup
- Water — 1 cup
- Pickling spices — 2 tsp
- Salt — 2 tsp + 1/8 tsp
- Red pepper flakes — 1/8 tsp
- Celery seeds — ½ tsp
- Lime beans, cooked — 1 1/2 cup
- Fresh tomatoes, diced — 2 cups
- Onion, diced — One
- Fresh cilantro — ¼ cup
- Salsa — Optional

Instructions:

1. Combine yogurt, curry powder, ginger, and lime juice. Coat chicken.
2. Marinate for 1 to 4 hours.

3. In a pan, mix vinegar and water and then add spices, 1/8 tsp salt, red pepper, and celery seeds. Boil and simmer for 5 mins.
4. Now add the lime beans and tomatoes with onions in a container and using a mesh sieve, pour the warm vinegar in the veggies. Add cilantro and let chill for 1 hour.
5. Remove chicken from marinade and season with remaining salt.
6. Place in on grill and cook for 8-10 mins.
7. Serve with salsa.

Baked Butternut Squash

"Enjoy flavors of this amazing baked dish that is easy to make and perfect side dish."

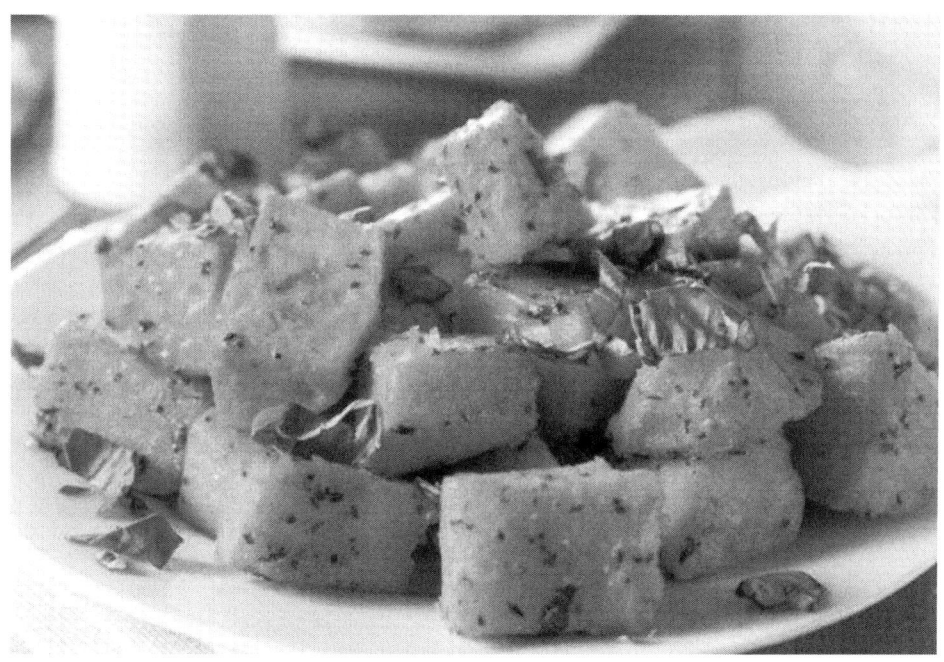

Prep Time:	10 minutes	Calories:	60
Cook Time:	30 minutes	Fat (g):	1g
Total Time:	40 minutes	Protein (g):	2g
Servings:	12	Net carbs:	11g

Ingredients:

- Large butternut squash   5 pounds
- Grounded cinnamon   ¼ tsp
- Salt   1/8 tsp
- Black pepper   1/8 tsp

Instructions:

1. Preheat oven to 350 F.
2. Remove the seeds from squash and cut it in large cubes.
3. Mix in the cinnamon, salt, and pepper and place on a baking sheet and bake for 30-35 minutes.
4. Serve.

Baked Chicken Tenders

"Make these healthy and juicy chicken tenders in your kitchen and enjoy."

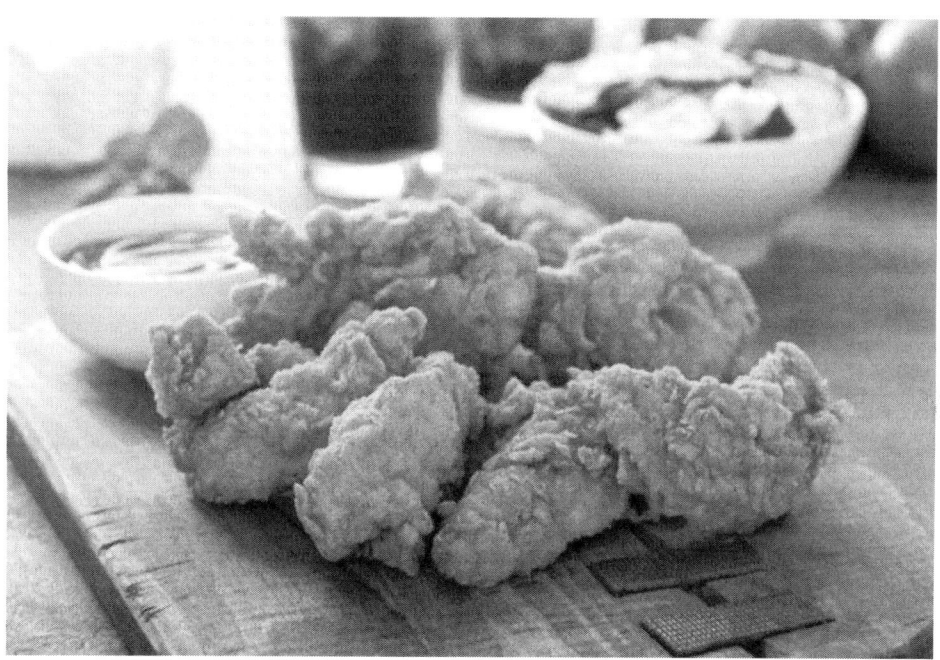

Prep Time:	15 minutes	Calories:	141
Cook Time:	15 minutes	Fat (g):	5g
Total Time:	30 minutes	Protein (g):	17g
Servings:	4	Net carbs:	6g

Ingredients:

- Chicken thighs — 1 pound
- Cornflake crumbs — 1 cup
- Italian herb seasoning — ½ tsp
- Garlic powder — ¼ tsp
- Onion powder — ¼ tsp
- Paprika — 1 tsp

Instructions:

1. Preheat oven to 400 F.
2. Cut chicken in bite-size pieces. In a plastic bag, crush the corn flakes and add in other ingredients. Shake until well-combined.
3. Add the chicken pieces in the bag and shake to coat well.
4. Spread the coated chicken pieces on a baking sheet and bake for 13-15 mins.
5. Serve immediately.

Panko and Parmesan Topped Zucchini

"Make these yummy appetizers in just a few minutes and enjoy good health."

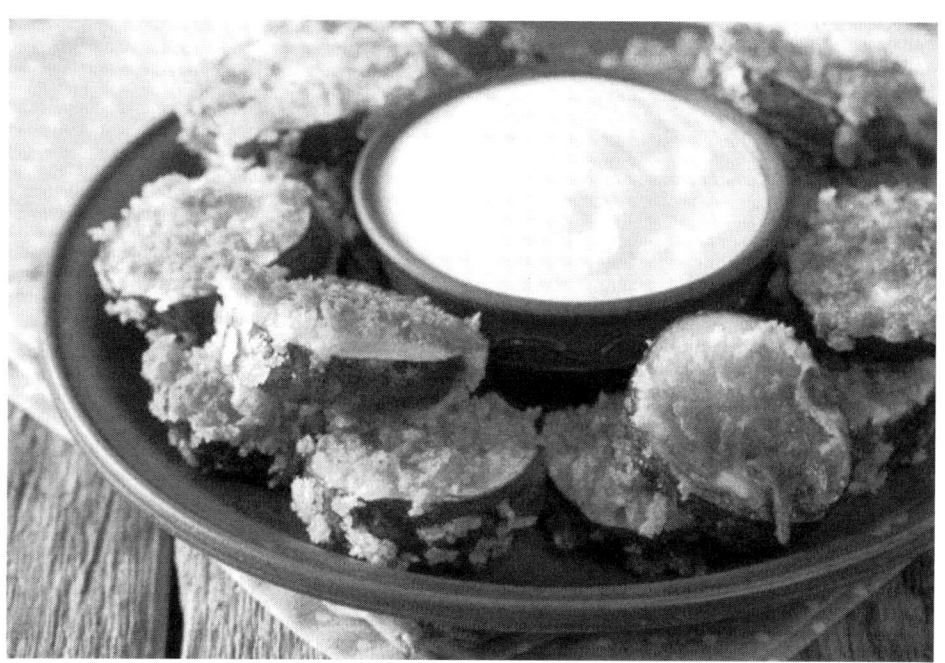

Prep Time:	20 minutes	Calories:	105
Cook Time:	30 minutes	Fat (g):	6g
Total Time:	50 minutes	Protein (g):	5g
Servings:	4	Net carbs:	8g

Ingredients:

- Zucchini — Two
- Panko breadcrumbs — 1/4 cup
- Grated parmesan — 1/4 cup
- Garlic powder — ½ tsp
- Onion powder — ½ tsp
- Salt — ¼ tsp
- Black pepper — ¼ tsp
- Reduced-fat mayonnaise — 1 tbsp

Instructions:

1. Preheat oven to 450 F. Slice the zucchini into rounds.
2. Mix all the topping ingredients.
3. Dip each round into the mixture, coating it evenly on both sides.
4. Bake the zucchini rounds for 20-25 minutes.
5. Serve immediately.

Veggie Burritos

"Stuff the tortillas with your desired veggies and fell in love with the taste of it."

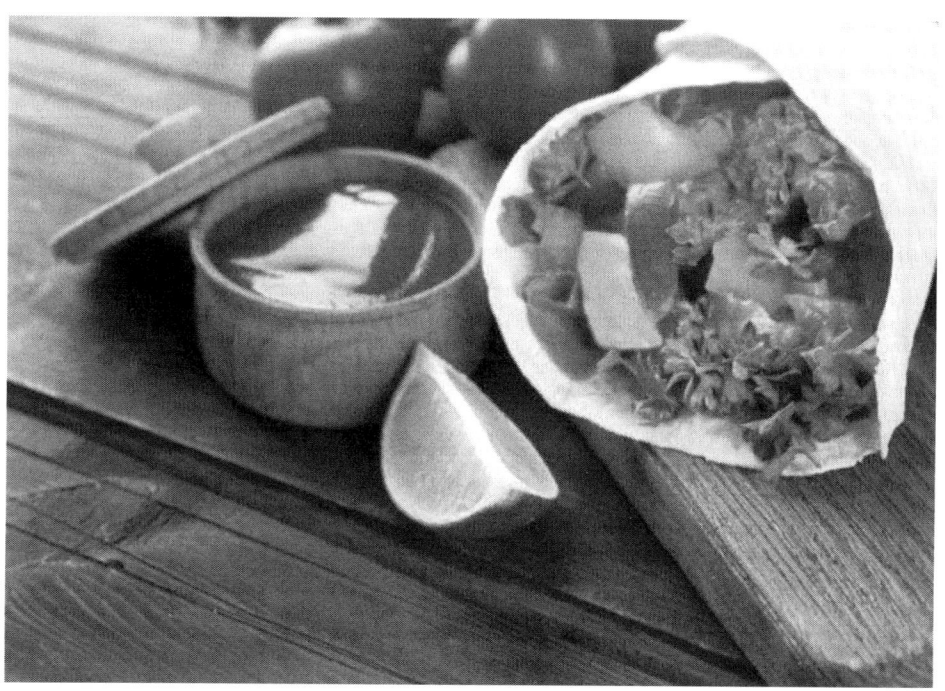

Prep Time:	10 minutes	Calories:	262
Cook Time:	25 minutes	Fat (g):	7g
Total Time:	35 minutes	Protein (g):	19g
Servings:	5	Net carbs:	46g

Ingredients:

- Vegetable oil — 1 tsp
- Onions, chopped — Two
- Garlic cloves, minced — Three
- Green bell pepper, chopped — One
- Zucchini, chopped — One
- Carrot, grated — One
- Chili powder — 2 tsp
- Dried oregano — 1 tsp
- Ground cumin — 1 tsp
- Salsa — 1 cup, divided
- Black beans, cooked — 16 ounces
- Flour tortillas — Five
- Shredded cheddar cheese — ½ cup

Instructions:

1. Preheat oven to 400 F.
2. Cook onions in oil in a pan and then add in green pepper, garlic, zucchini, and carrot and cook for 3-4 mins. Add oregano, cumin, and chili powder.
3. Remove from heat and add in half of salsa and beans and spoon over the tortillas. Fold the tortilla and place seam side down with remaining salsa.
4. Bake for 15 mins then sprinkle cheese and bake for the other 5 mins. Serve.

Beef and Zucchini Meatballs

"This is the best combination ever to make some healthy and perfect meatballs."

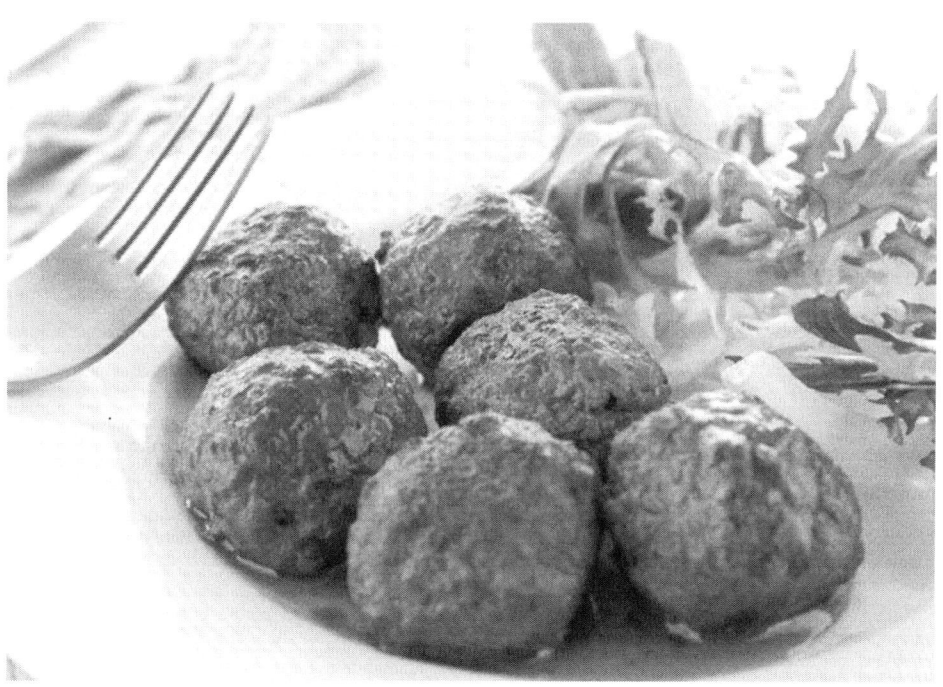

Prep Time:	5 minutes	Calories:	397
Cook Time:	25 minutes	Fat (g):	24g
Total Time:	30 minutes	Protein (g):	36g
Servings:	4	Net carbs:	4g

Ingredients:

- Ground beef — 1 pound
- Grated zucchini — 1 cup
- Salt — ¼ tsp
- Pepper — ¼ tsp

Instructions:

1. Preheat oven to 400 F.
2. In a bowl, mix all ingredients and shape in 20 meatballs.
3. Place on a baking sheet and bake for 23-25 mins.
4. Serve hot.

Roasted Chickpeas

"Roast chickpeas and satisfy your mid-day cravings in the best way."

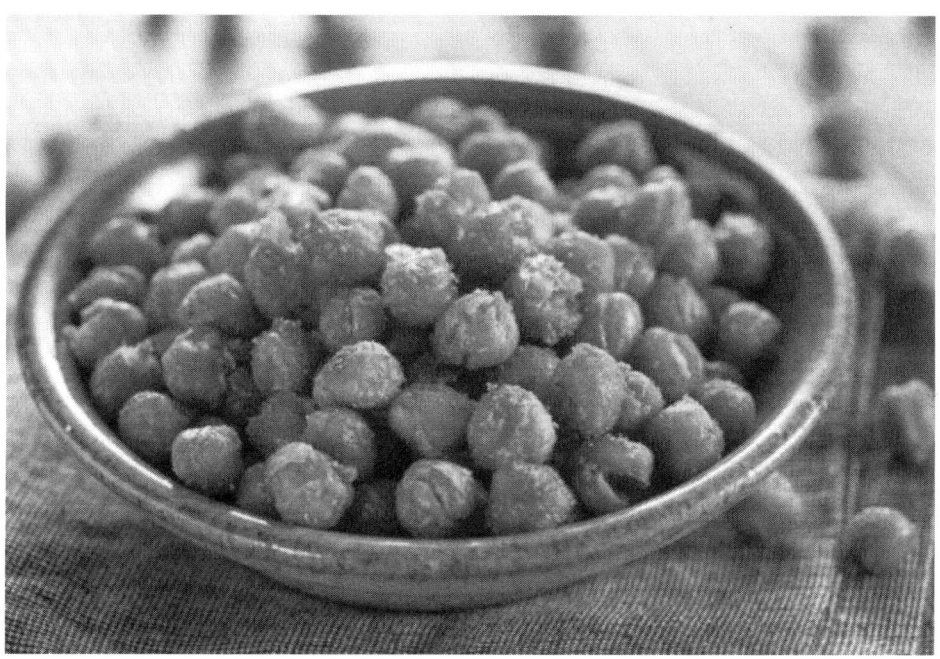

Prep Time:	1 minute	Calories:	105
Cook Time:	44 minutes	Fat (g):	3g
Total Time:	45 minutes	Protein (g):	3g
Servings:	4	Net carbs:	16g

Ingredients:

- Chickpeas — 15 ounces
- Olive oil — 2 tsp
- Salt and pepper — To taste

Instructions:

1. Preheat oven to 425 F.
2. Spread beans on a baking sheet and bake for 22 minutes.
3. Take out, sprinkle oil, pepper, and salt and bake more for 22 more minutes.
4. Serve.

Meatballs with Spaghetti

"Meatballs with spaghetti is everyone's favorite comfort food, and in this recipe you can make it if you are following the diabetic diet."

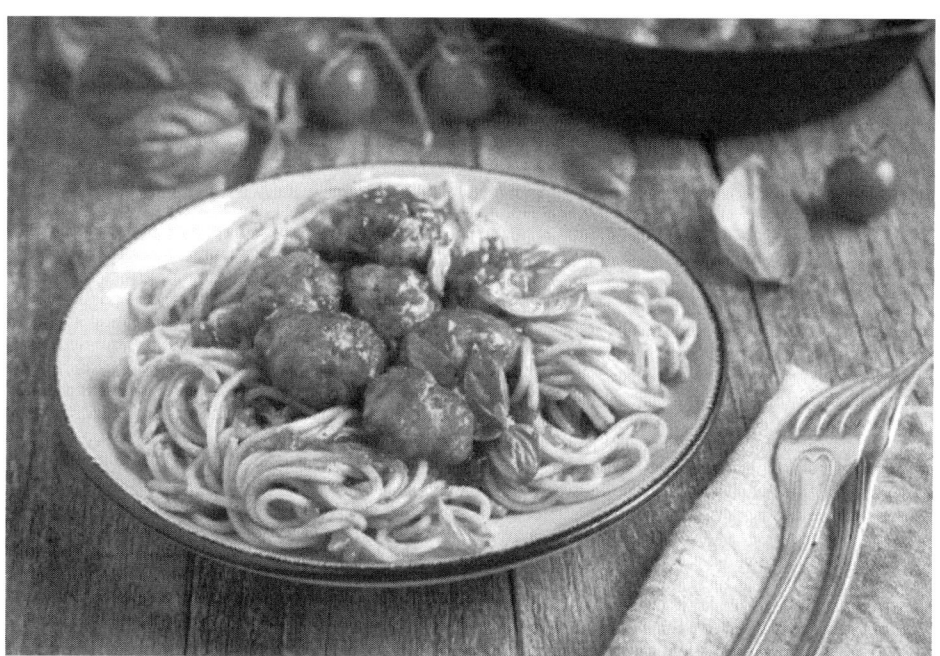

Prep Time:	15 minutes	Calories:	381
Cook Time:	30 minutes	Fat (g):	11g
Total Time:	45 minutes	Protein (g):	25g
Servings:	6	Net carbs:	48g

Ingredients:

- Grounded turkey breast — 1 pound
- Chopped onion — ½ cup
- Egg, beaten — One
- Plain bread crumbs — ¼ cup
- Garlic powder — 1 tsp
- Salt — ½ tsp
- Black pepper — ½ tsp
- Canola oil — 1 tbsp
- Sliced mushrooms — 8 ounces
- Marinara sauce — 26 ounces
- Spaghetti — 12 ounces
- Dried basil leaves — ½ tsp

Instructions:

1. Combine turkey with onions, breadcrumbs, eggs, salt, pepper, and garlic powder. Mix well and form in meatballs.
2. In a skillet, cook meatballs and remove them. Then cook mushrooms and add in marinara and basil. Add in meatballs and cook for 11-12 mins.
3. Serve with spaghetti.

Lasagna Rolls

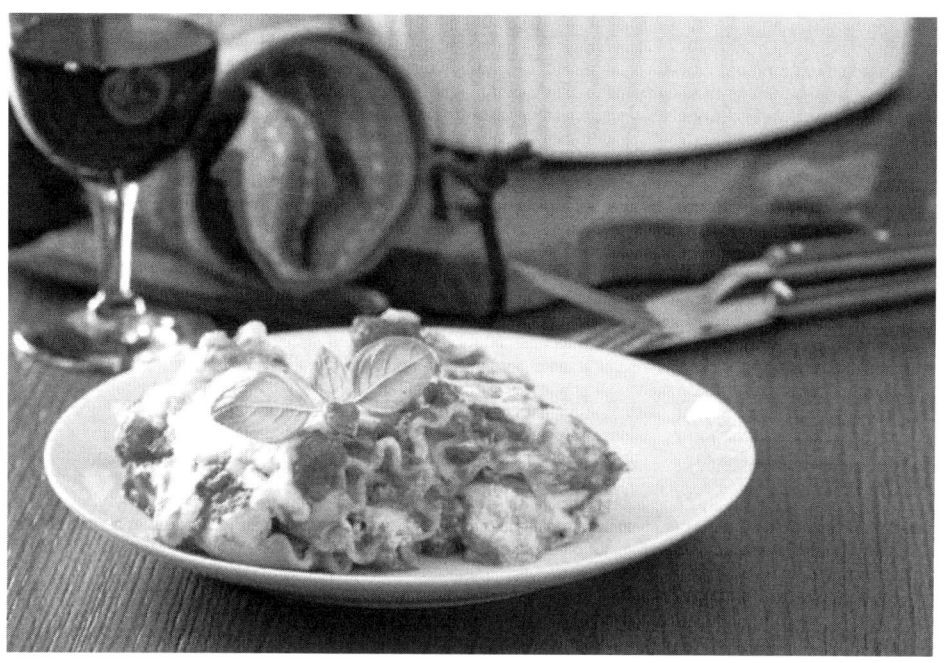

Prep Time:	5 minutes	**Calories:**	188
Cook Time:	50 minutes	**Fat (g):**	9g
Total Time:	55 minutes	**Protein (g):**	14g
Servings:	10	**Net carbs:**	13g

Ingredients:

- Olive oil — 2 tsp
- Chopped onions — ½ cup
- Tomato and basil sauce — 24 ounces
- Ricotta cheese — 1 cup
- Egg substitute — ¼ cup
- Minced garlic cloves — Three
- Artichoke hearts, quartered — 14 ounce
- Fresh chopped basil — 2 tbsp
- Parmesan cheese, grated — 2 tbsp
- Lasagna noodles, cooked — Ten

Instructions:

1. Preheat oven to 350 F.
2. Heat oil in a pan and sauté onions in it. Add in tomato sauce and cook and add the 1 cup sauce in a baking dish.
3. In a bowl combine the ricotta, eggs, artichoke hearts, garlic, basil, and parmesan. Spoon the mixture over the noodles and roll-up. Place in the baking dish and top with tomato sauce and bake covered for 42-45 mins.

Lentil Soup

"This is the simplest way to make this easy and yummy lentil soup. It is really fast and easy to make."

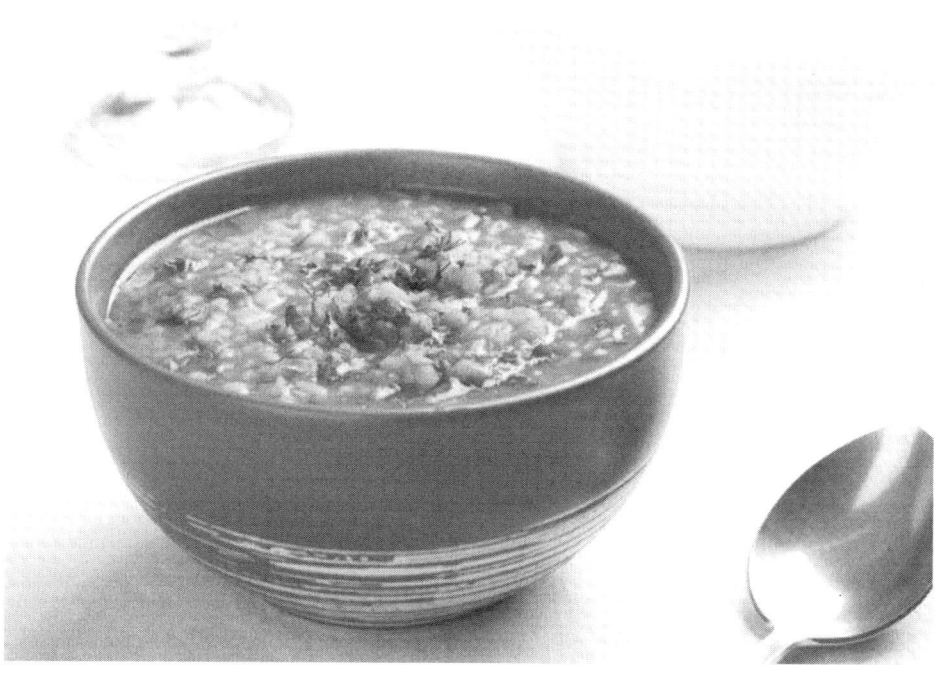

Prep Time:	5 minutes	Calories:	115
Cook Time:	55 minutes	Fat (g):	7g
Total Time:	60 minutes	Protein (g):	8g
Servings:	8	Net carbs:	20g

Ingredients:

- Chopped onion — 1 cup
- Red or green bell pepper, chopped — 1 cup
- Celery, chopped — 1 cup
- Carrots, chopped — 1 cup
- Brown lentils — 1 cup
- Dried oregano — 1 tsp
- Water — 3 cups
- Beef broth — 3 cups
- Garlic powder — 1 tsp
- Salt — ½ tsp
- Pepper — ½ tsp

Instructions:

1. Cook onions, bell peppers, celery, and carrots in a soup pot.
2. Add the remaining ingredients after 8-10 mins.
3. Bring to boil and then cook for 55-60 mins on low heat.
4. Serve.

Irish Beef Pot Pie

"This is the yummy and delicious beef pie with fried carrots and pies. You can add in any vegetables of your preference."

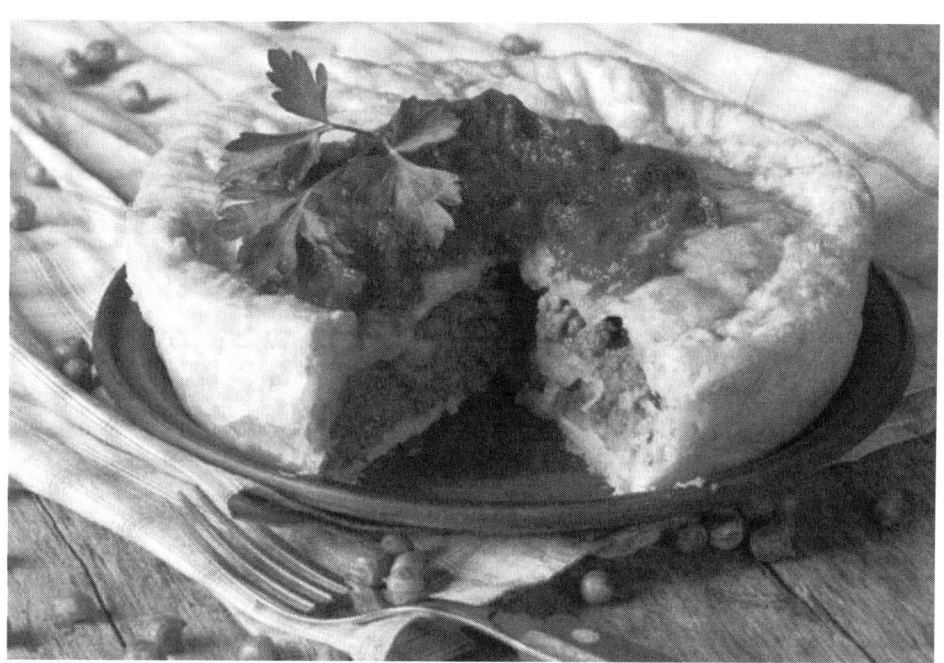

Prep Time:	10 minutes	Calories:	402
Cook Time:	30 minutes	Fat (g):	18g
Total Time:	40 minutes	Protein (g):	27g
Servings:	6	Net carbs:	31g

Ingredients:

- Beef flat iron steaks — 1 ½ pound
- Cremini mushrooms, sliced — 8 ounces
- Frozen Sliced carrots — 1 ½ cup
- Frozen peas — 1 ½ cup
- Fresh thyme, chopped — 2 tsp, divided
- Minced garlic — 1 tsp, divided
- Salt and pepper — To taste
- Cornstarch — 3 tbsp
- Beef broth — 14 ounces
- Refrigerated pie crust — 7 ounces

Instructions:

1. Preheat oven to 425 F.
2. Cut the steaks in strips. In a skillet, add the mushrooms and cook for 3 mins.
3. Add in carrots, peas, thyme, and garlic and cook for 4-5 mins. Remove from skillet and add beef in the skillet and cook for 2 mins.
4. Season with salt and pepper and take out. Now mix cornstarch in the broth and cook in the same skillet until slightly thick. Add in beef and veggies.
5. Place the beef mixture in a pie plate and place the crust on the mixture and bake for 19-20 mins. Serve when done.

Vanilla French Toast

"This vanilla French toast is the best thing to add in your breakfast or brunch. It is easy to make and totally sugar-free."

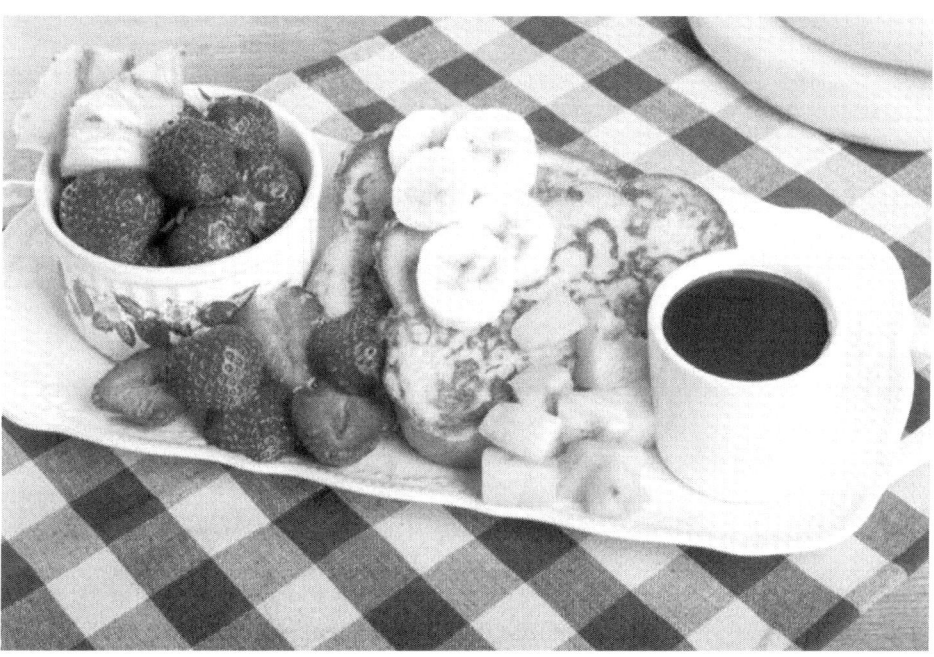

Prep Time:	5 minutes	Calories:	100
Cook Time:	5 minutes	Fat (g):	3g
Total Time:	10 minutes	Protein (g):	6g
Servings:	6	Net carbs:	11g

Ingredients:

- Large eggs — Two
- Milk — ½ cup
- Vanilla extract — ½ tsp
- Whole wheat bread — 6 slices
- Grounded cinnamon — 1/8 tsp
- Bananas and berries, optional

Instructions:

1. Preheat pan on medium heat.
2. Beat the eggs with milk and vanilla together and add in cinnamon.
3. Grease pan with oil and dip the bread slices in the egg mixture and coat from both sides.
4. Cook from both sides until golden brown.
5. The delicious toast is ready.

Reuben Sandwich

"This classic and yummy Reuben sandwich is a perfect appetizer and tastes terrific."

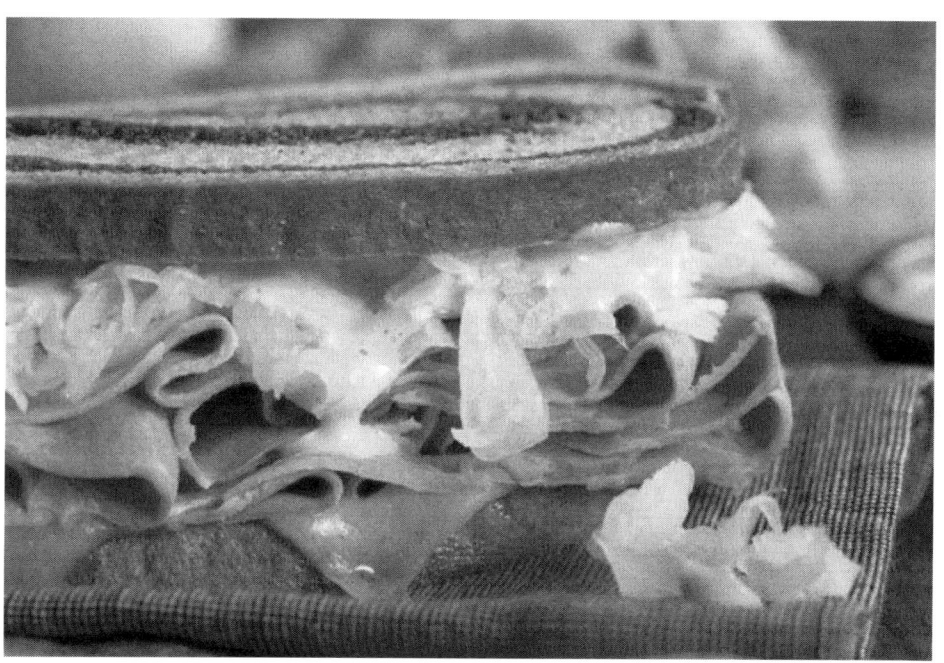

Prep Time:	10 minutes	**Calories:**	414
Cook Time:	15 minutes	**Fat (g):**	16g
Total Time:	25 minutes	**Protein (g):**	32g
Servings:	4	**Net carbs:**	41g

Ingredients:

- Thin sliced deli corned beef — 12 ounces
- Thousand Island dressing — ½ cup, divided
- Rye bread — 8 slices
- Swiss cheese — 8 slices
- Drained sauerkraut — 1 cup

Instructions:

1. Preheat oven to 425 F.
2. Spread 2 tsp of dressing on bread slices and cut in quarters.
3. Place the slices on a baking sheet and bake for 9-10 mins.
4. Cut cheese slices in quarters.
5. Top the bread slices with corned beef, cheese slices, and sauerkraut.
6. Bake for 4-5 mins on 425 F until cheese melts. Top with dressing and serve.

Mashed Potatoes

"This mashed potatoes dish is made from cauliflowers and is all-time favorite comfort food."

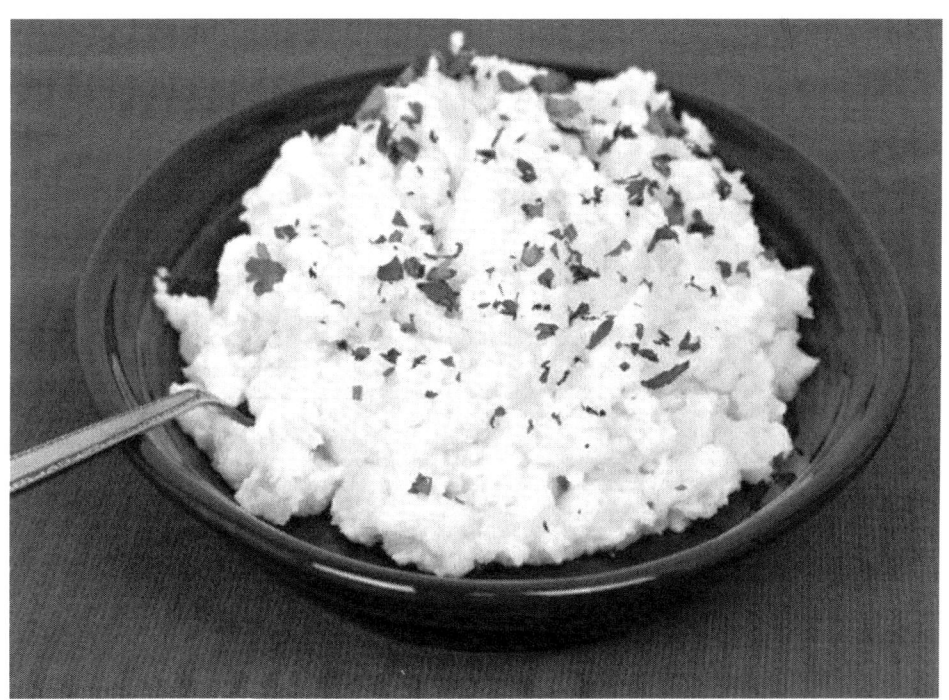

Prep Time:	10 minutes	**Calories:**	87
Cook Time:	15 minutes	**Fat (g):**	5g
Total Time:	25 minutes	**Protein (g):**	3g
Servings:	4	**Net carbs:**	7g

Ingredients:

- Cauliflower — One
- Green onions, sliced — Four
- Garlic cloves — Four
- Unsweetened almond milk — ¼ cup
- Extra virgin olive oil — 4 tsp
- Black pepper — To taste
- Chopped chives — 1 tbsp

Instructions:

1. Put the cauliflower, onions, and garlic in a steamer and steam for a maximum of 15 minutes. Add in a blender and blend well.
2. Add in milk and 2 tbsp oil and blend again.
3. Season with salt and pepper. Garnish with remaining oil and chives. Serve.

Lemon Herb Pot Roast

"Making this pot roast is a perfect and easy homemade dish. You can combine it with any veggies of your desire."

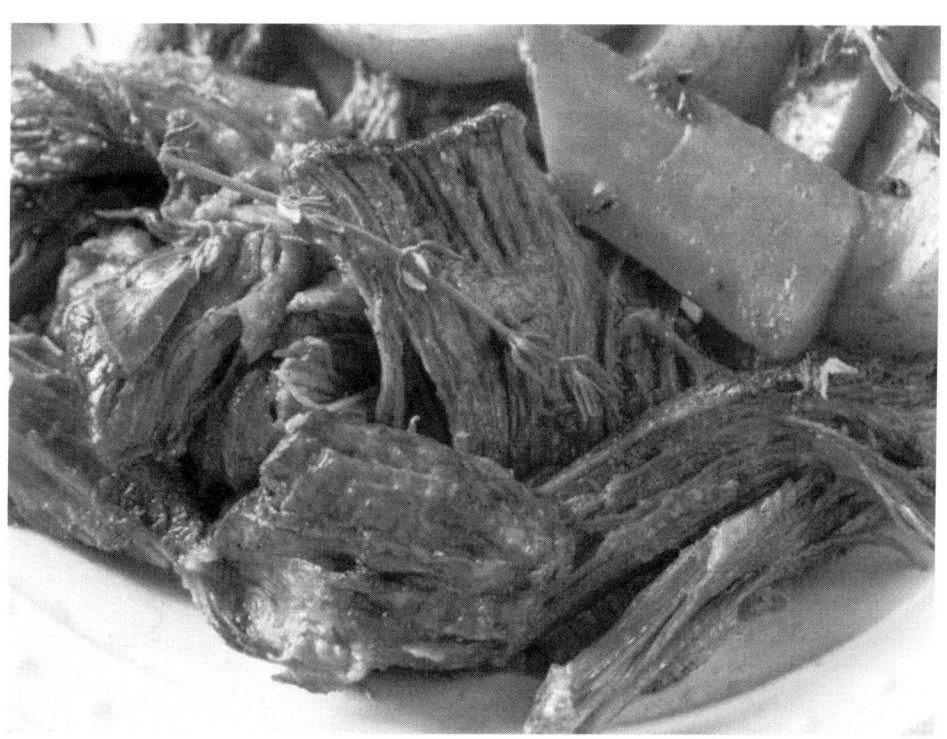

Prep Time:	5 minutes	Calories:	335
Cook Time:	3 hours	Fat (g):	11g
Total Time:	3 hour 5 minutes	Protein (g):	36g
Servings:	6	Net carbs:	18g

Ingredients:

- Beef shoulder roast — 2 ½ pound
- Olive oil — 1 tbsp
- Baby carrots — 2 cups
- Potato wedges — 1 pound
- Onion wedges — Six
- Cornstarch dissolved in 2 tbsp water — 2 tbsp
- Basil seasoning — ½ tsp
- Lemon pepper — 2 tsp
- Minced garlic — Two cloves
- Dried basil — 1 tsp

Instructions:

1. Combine the seasoning ingredients and press on beef.
2. Heat oil in Dutch oven and then brown the pot roast. Add 1 cup of water and bring to a boil.
3. Reduce heat and cook for 2 hours. Add veggies and cook for 45 more mins.
4. Add cornstarch and cook until thick.
5. Serve.

Lima Beans

"These lime beans are super easy to make at home, enjoy the best diabetic dish."

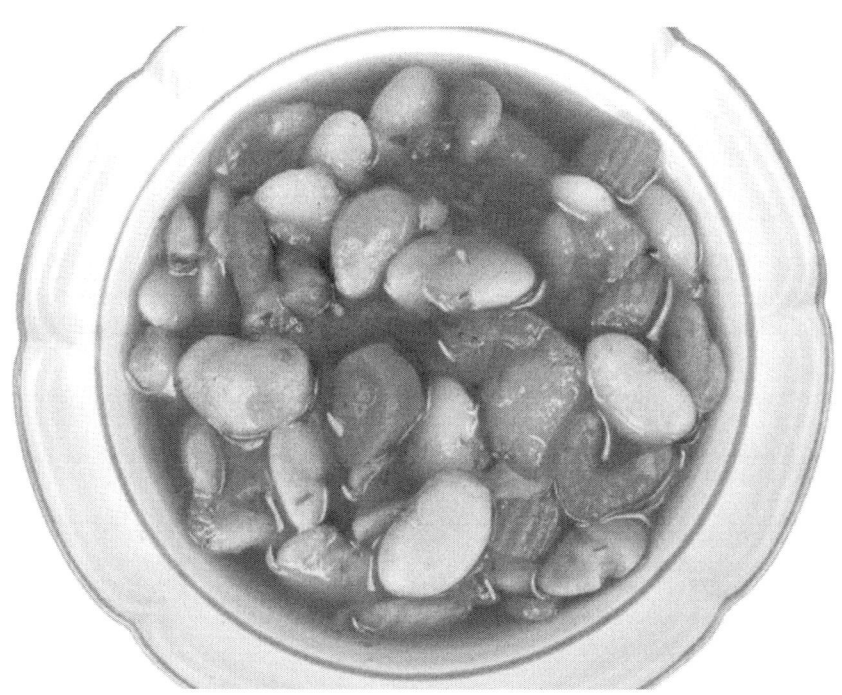

Prep Time:	5 minutes	Calories:	84
Cook Time:	35 minutes	Fat (g):	0g
Total Time:	40 minutes	Protein (g):	4g
Servings:	6	Net carbs:	15g

Ingredients:

- Chopped onion   Half
- Chicken broth   1 ½ cup
- Lima beans   16 ounces
- Cooking spray

Instructions:

1. Heat the saucepan and grease with cooking spray. Sauté the onions and when translucent, add in broth and bring to a boil.
2. Add lima beans in boiled broth.
3. Reduce heat and cook for 30 minutes or until beans are tender.

Oats and Quinoa Breakfast

"Enjoy breakfast with oats and quinoa, and keep yourself healthy and smart."

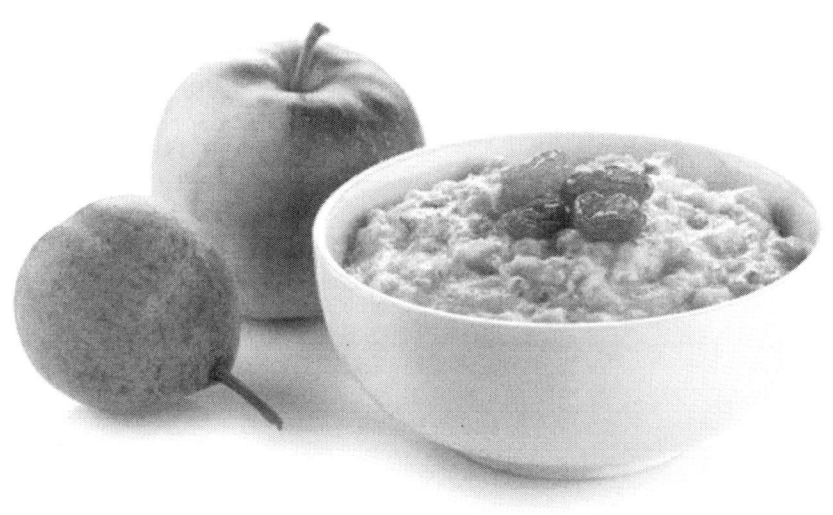

Prep Time:	10 minutes	Calories:	191
Cook Time:	20 minutes	Fat (g):	4g
Total Time:	30 minutes	Protein (g):	7g
Servings:	4	Net carbs:	30g

Ingredients:

- Quinoa — ½ cup
- Steel-cut oats — ½ cup
- Water — 3 cups
- Almond meal — 2 tbsp
- Flaxseeds meals — 2 tbsp
- Ground cinnamon — 1 tbsp

Instructions:

1. Boil water in a pot and add oats and quinoa in it.
2. Cook until quinoa is tender.
3. Add in almond and flaxseed meal and serve with cinnamon topping.

Avocado Toast

"Top your bread slices with mashed avocados with a lemon twist and have a nice day ahead."

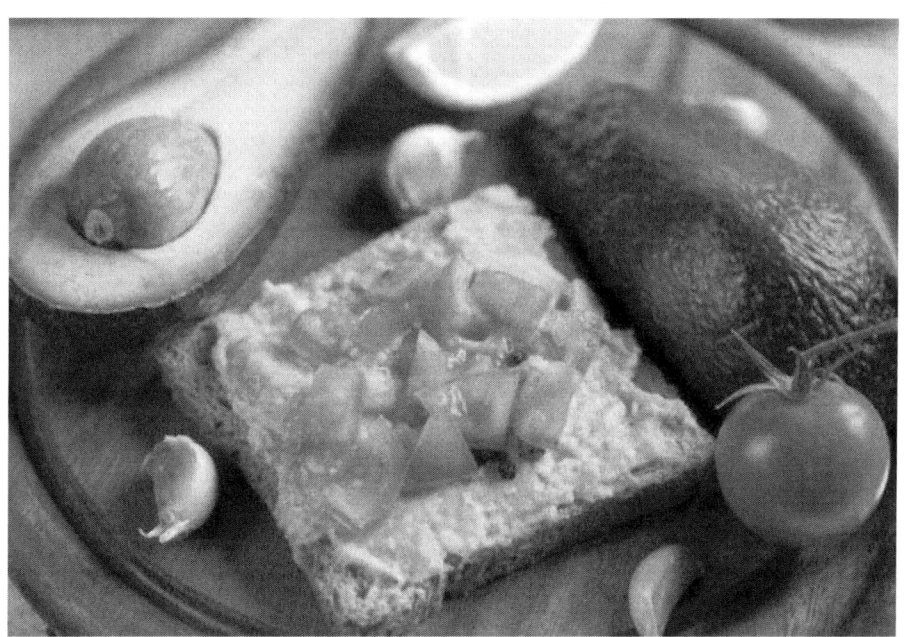

Prep Time:	10 minutes	Calories:	72
Cook Time:	5 minutes	Fat (g):	1g
Total Time:	15 minutes	Protein (g):	3g
Servings:	2	Net carbs:	11g

Ingredients:

- Whole grain bread — 2 slices
- Avocado — Half
- Chopped cilantro — 2 tbsp
- Lemon juice — 1 tsp
- Lemon zest — ¼ tsp
- Cayenne pepper — A pinch
- Salt — A pinch
- Chia seeds — ¼ tsp

Instructions:

1. Toast the bread slices for 3 minutes.
2. Mash avocado in a bowl then mix in cilantro, lemon juice, lemon zest, cayenne, and salt.
3. Spread on slices and sprinkle chia seeds. Serve.

Bean Soup with Kale

"Beans lover should never miss out on this amazing recipe of bean soup with kale."

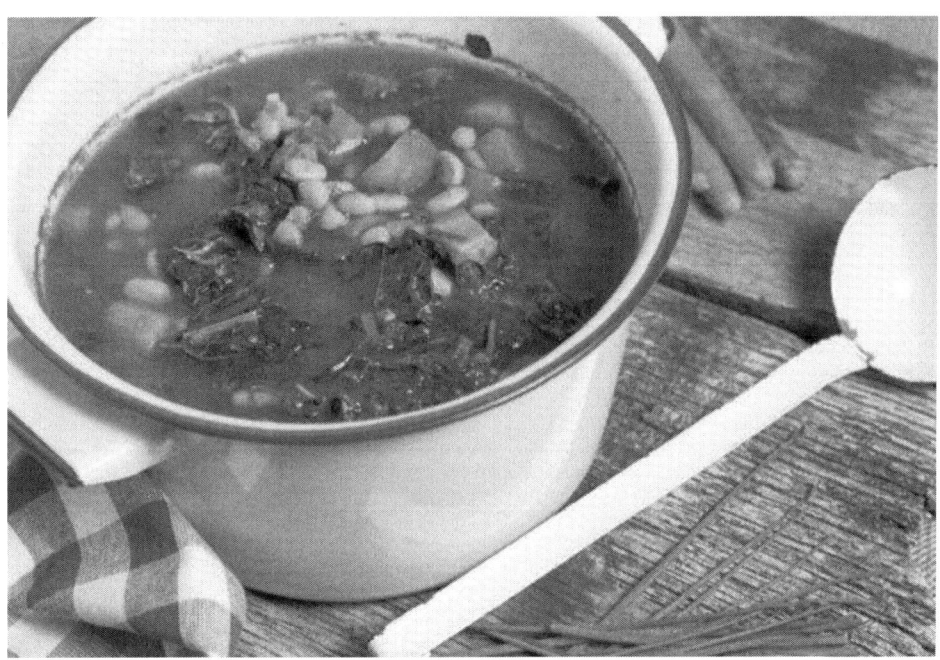

Prep Time:	10 minutes	Calories:	182
Cook Time:	30 minutes	Fat (g):	2g
Total Time:	40 minutes	Protein (g):	11g
Servings:	8	Net carbs:	31g

Ingredients:

- Olive oil — 1 tbsp
- Garlic cloves, minced — Eight
- Yellow onion, chopped — One
- Raw kale, chopped — 4 cups
- Chicken or vegetable broth — 4 cups
- Cooked white beans — 15 ounces
- Plum tomatoes, chopped — Four
- Italian herb seasoning — 2 tsp
- Salt and pepper — To taste
- Chopped parsley — 1 cup

Instructions:

1. Heat oil in a pan and sauté onions and garlic in it. Add kale and cook.
2. Now add in 3 cups of broth with 2 cups of beans and also add tomatoes, Italian seasoning, salt, and pepper and cook it for 5 mins.
3. Blend the remaining broth and beans in a food processor and add in the soup. Cook on low heat for 13-15 mins. Garnish with parsley and serve.

Stir-fried Chicken

"This diabetic-friendly dish is easy to make and really quick."

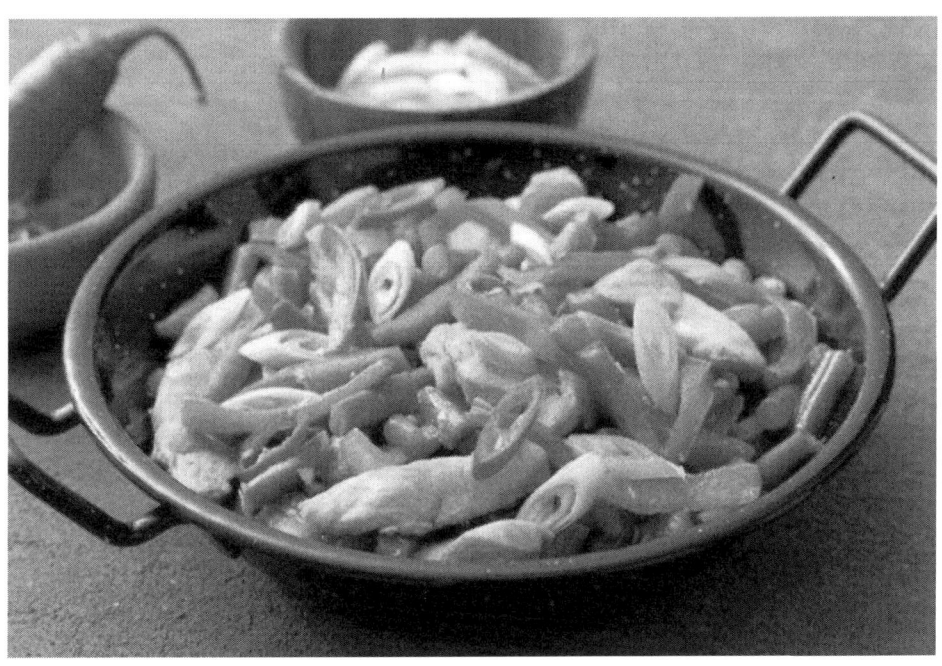

Prep Time:	10 minutes	**Calories:**	258
Cook Time:	15 minutes	**Fat (g):**	8g
Total Time:	25 minutes	**Protein (g):**	38g
Servings:	4	**Net carbs:**	6g

Ingredients:

- Canola oil — 3 tsp, divided
- Boneless chicken strips — 1 ½ pound
- Garlic cloves, minced — Four
- Asparagus — 8 ounces
- Red bell pepper — Half
- Grated ginger — 1 tbsp
- Chicken broth — ½ cup
- Soy sauce — 2 tbsp
- Water — 2 tbsp
- Black pepper — ½ tsp
- Cornstarch — 2 tsp

Instructions:

1. In a pan, add 2 tsp oil and cook chicken with garlic for 5 mins. Remove chicken.
2. Add 1 tsp oil and cook asparagus, bell pepper, and ginger for 4 mins.
3. Combine chicken broth with soy sauce, water, and black pepper in a bowl.
4. Add in cornstarch and mix. Add it in vegetables and cook 1 minute.
5. Add in chicken and cook for a couple of mins and serve.

Cheesy Quesadillas

"This quesadillas recipe includes black beans and your favorite cheese to enjoy a healthy breakfast."

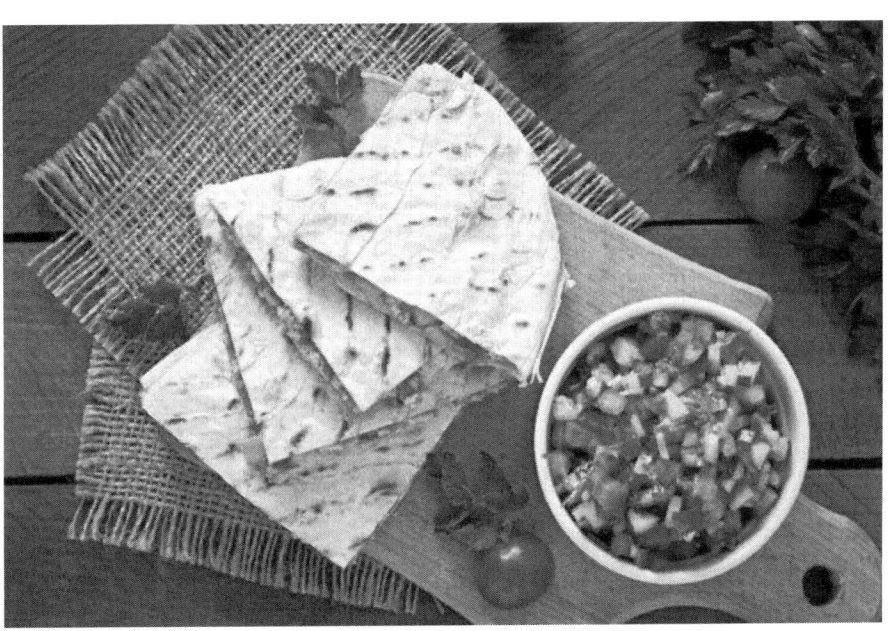

Prep Time:	10 minutes	**Calories:**	125
Cook Time:	5 minutes	**Fat (g):**	5g
Total Time:	15 minutes	**Protein (g):**	12g
Servings:	12	**Net carbs:**	21g

Ingredients:

- Black beans, cooked — 1 cup
- Mild salsa — 1 cup, divided
- Cumin — 1 tsp
- Whole wheat tortilla — Twelve
- Shredded Jack cheese — 1 cup
- Scallions — ¼ cup
- Fresh cilantro — 1 tbsp

Instructions:

1. Mash beans with a fork and add in ¼ cup of salsa and cumin.
2. Spoon the mixture evenly on 6 tortillas and sprinkle cheese, scallion, and cilantro. Top with remaining tortillas.
3. In a pan, cook quesadillas for 2-3 mins. Flip and cook from another side for 2 mins. Do with remaining quesadillas and cut in wedges.

Cucumber Salad

"Make this cucumber salad in your favorite dressing and enjoy good diabetic food."

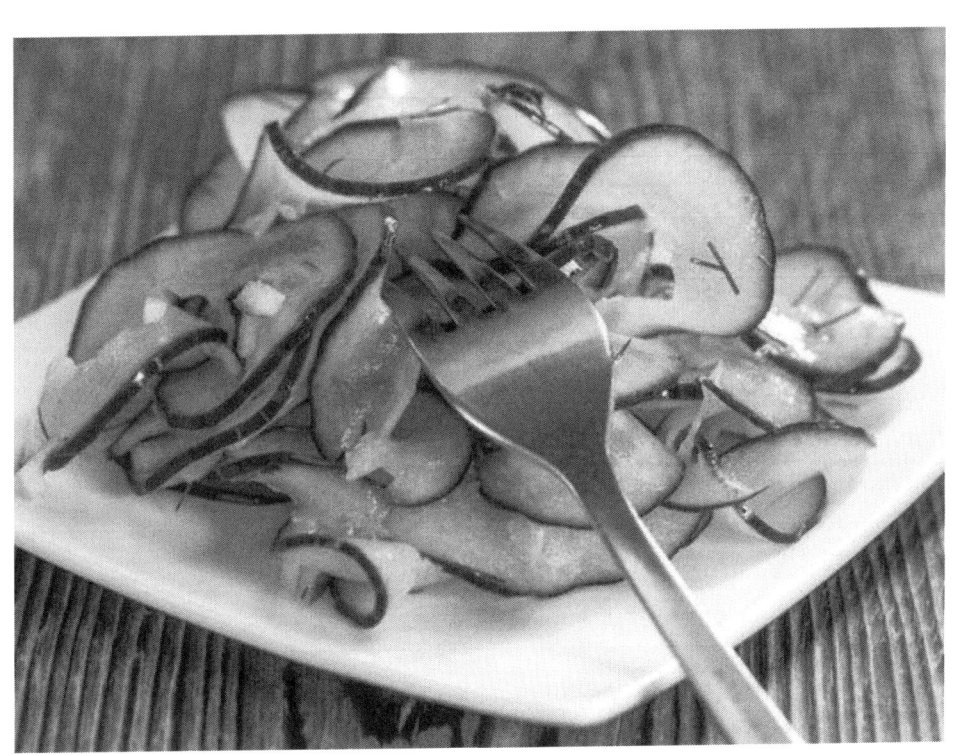

Prep Time:	10 minutes	Calories:	49
Cook Time:	0 minutes	Fat (g):	2g
Total Time:	10 minutes	Protein (g):	1g
Servings:	4	Net carbs:	5g

Ingredients:

- Fat-free French dressing — ¼ cup
- Fat-free mayonnaise — 1 tbsp
- Chopped parsley — 2 tbsp
- White vinegar — 1 tbsp
- Garlic, chopped — 1 tsp
- Salt — ½ tsp
- Sliced cucumbers — 2 ¼ cups
- Chopped onions — ¼ cup

Instructions:

1. In a bowl, mix French dressing with mayonnaise, vinegar, garlic, salt, and parsley.
2. Add in cucumbers and onions and let chill. Serve.

Beef Macaroni

"Have the benefits of this beefy macaroni when you are following a full diabetic diet."

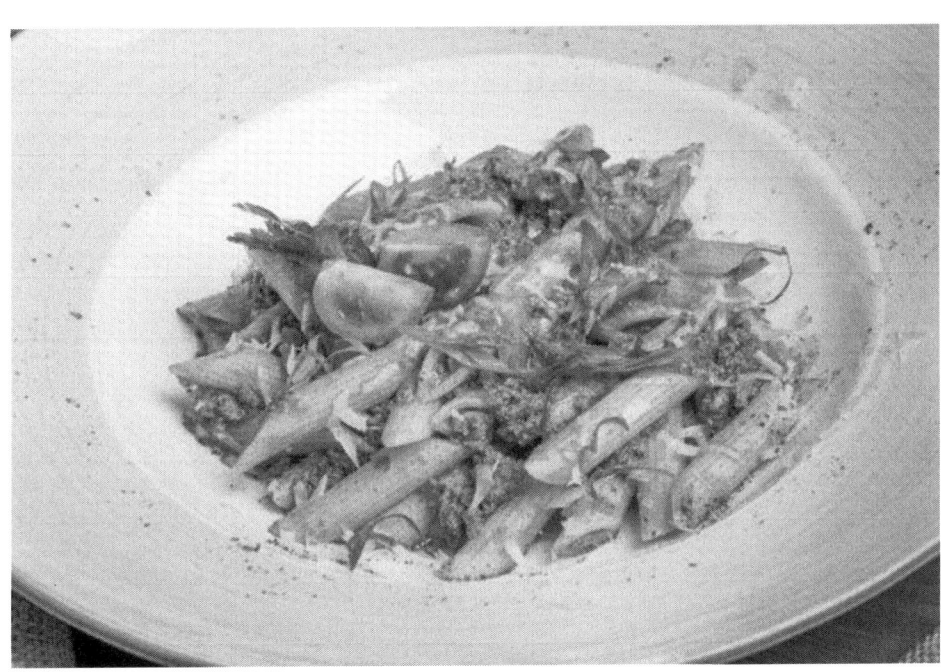

Prep Time:	5 minutes	Calories:	358
Cook Time:	20 minutes	Fat (g):	9g
Total Time:	25 minutes	Protein (g):	22g
Servings:	6	Net carbs:	49g

Ingredients:

- Extra-lean grounded beef — 1 pound
- Onion, chopped — One
- Water — 3 cups
- Whole kernel corns — 15 ounces
- Diced tomatoes — 14 ounces
- Taco seasoning mix — 1 ounce
- Low-carb pasta — 8 ounces

Instructions:

1. In a pot, cook beef and onion for 8-10 mins. Add water with corn, taco seasoning, and tomatoes. Mix.
2. Bring to a boil and add in pasta and cook for 10-12 mins on low heat. Serve.

Roasted Briskets

"Roast briskets and enjoy with your favorite dip or chutney."

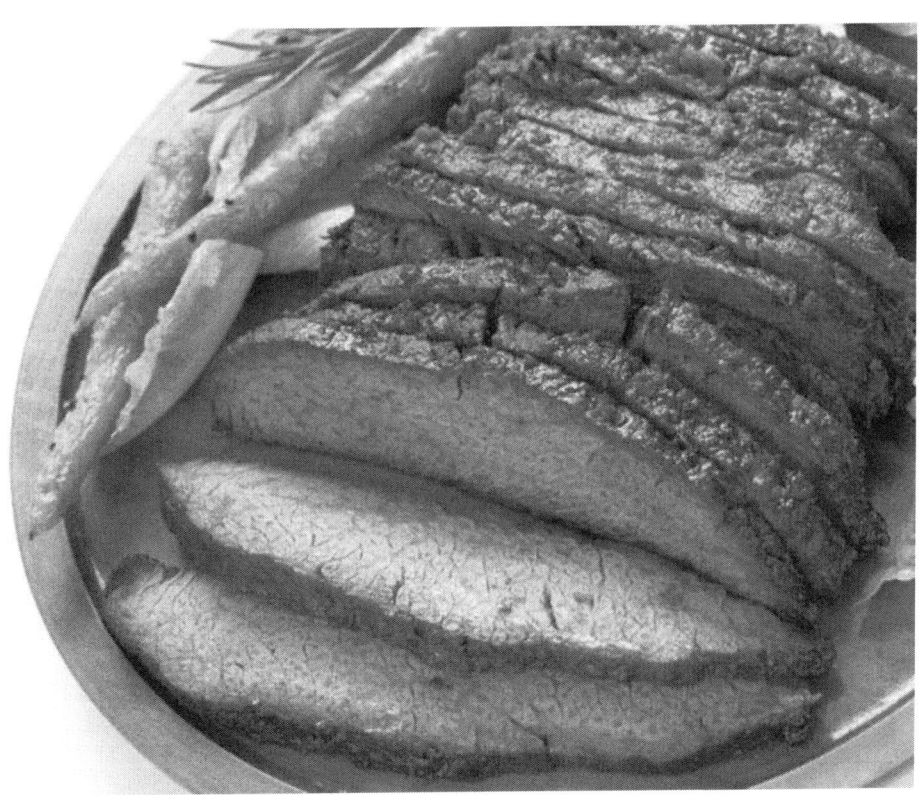

Prep Time:	10 minutes	Calories:	337
Cook Time:	3 hours	Fat (g):	17g
Total Time:	3 hours 10 minutes	Protein (g):	39g
Servings:	10	Net carbs:	4g

Ingredients:

- Fresh beef brisket — 4 pounds
- Small onions, quartered — Three
- Fresh mushrooms, halves — 1 pound
- Garlic cloves — Ten
- Water — 2 cups
- Tomato paste — 6 ounces
- Salt — 2 ½ tsp
- Black pepper — ¾ tsp

Instructions:

1. Preheat oven to 350 F.
2. Place brisket in roasting pan and set aside.
3. In a bowl, combine the onions, garlic, mushrooms, tomato paste, water, salt, and pepper. Pour over meat.
4. Cover it with aluminum foil and cook for 3 hours.
5. Slice it and cook for five more mins and serve.

Veggie Stuffed Pita

"This whole wheat pita bread can be filled with your favorite diabetic vegetables to give you a perfectly healthy diet."

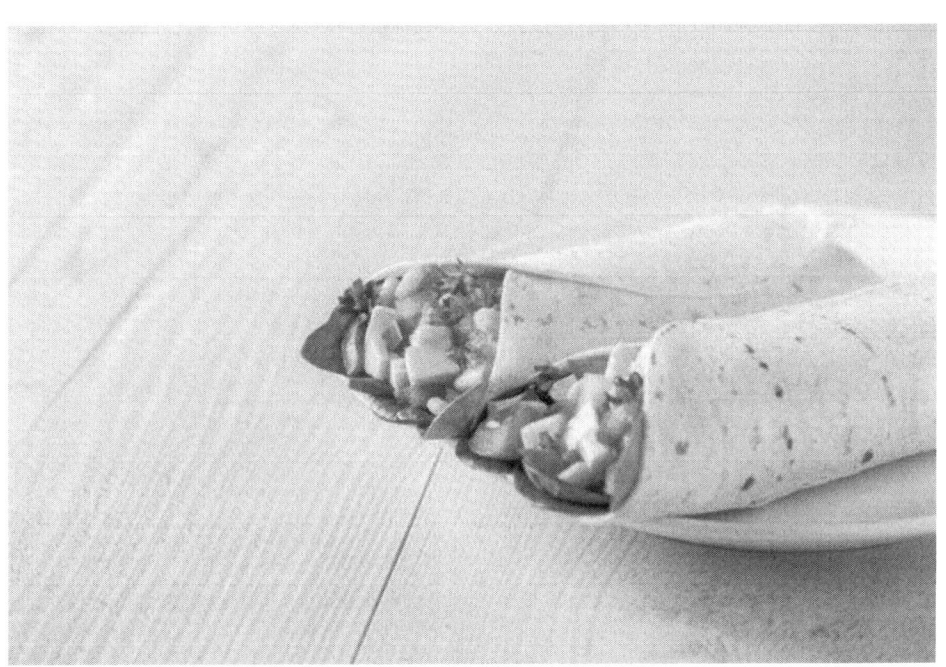

Prep Time:	5 minutes	Calories:	66
Cook Time:	0 minutes	Fat (g):	13g
Total Time:	5 minutes	Protein (g):	2g
Servings:	4	Net carbs:	12g

Ingredients:

- Shredded iceberg lettuce   4 cups
- Roma tomatoes, chopped   ½ cup
- Chopped cucumber   ½ cup
- Ranch dressing   2 tbsp
- Whole wheat pita bread, half   Two

Instructions:

1. Mix the lettuce, tomatoes, and cucumbers with dressing.
2. Open the bread halves and spoon mixture in each one of them.
3. Serve.

One-Pot Paella

"Cook rice with shrimps and turkey sausages and have a perfect and amazing fancy food."

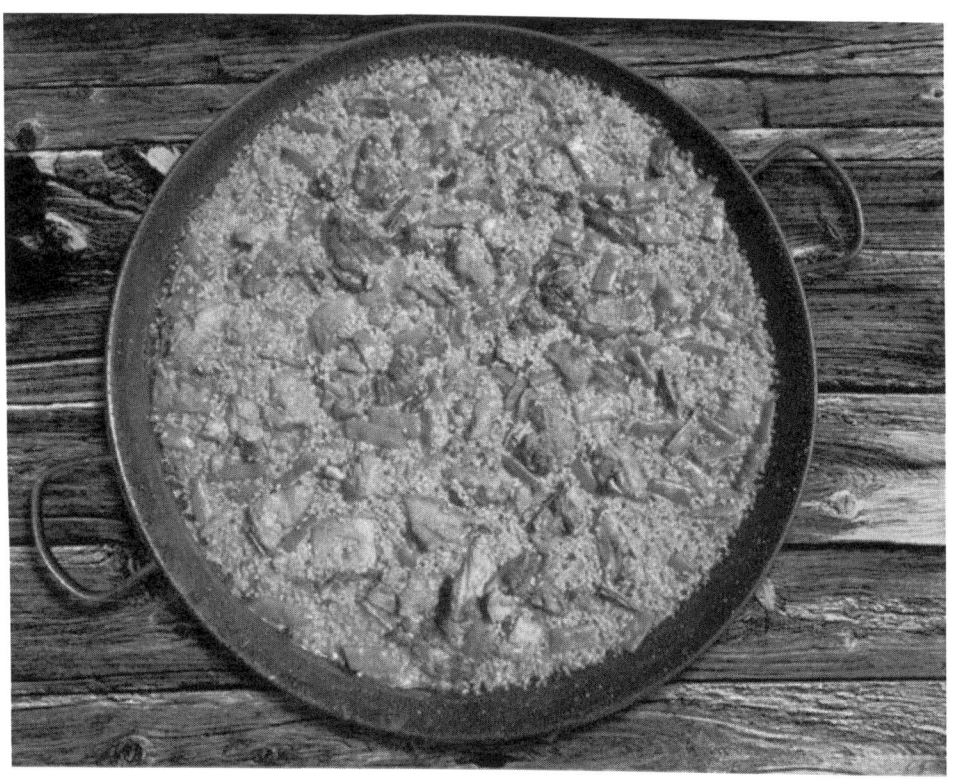

Prep Time:	10 minutes	**Calories:**	200
Cook Time:	35 minutes	**Fat (g):**	4g
Total Time:	45 minutes	**Protein (g):**	20g
Servings:	6	**Net carbs:**	30g

Ingredients:

- Turkey sausage — Half pound
- Onion, chopped — One
- Red bell pepper — One
- Garlic cloves, minced — Three
- Dried thyme — 1 tsp
- Uncooked cauliflower rice — 1 ½ cup
- Water — ¾ cup
- Diced tomatoes — 15 ounces
- Clam juice — 8 ounces
- Ground turmeric — ½ tsp
- Shrimps — ½ pound

Instructions:

1. Cook turkey sausage in a pot for 4-5 mins.
2. Add in onions, bell peppers, thyme, and garlic. Cook for 4-5 mins.
3. Add the cauliflower rice, tomatoes, water, and juice with turmeric and mix well.
4. Bring to a boil and cook 20 mins on low heat.
5. Add in shrimps and cook for 5 mins until the rice is tender. Serve.

Comfort Shepherd's Pie

"This Shepherd's pie is not just your regular pie. It is made of some amazing and healthy ingredients."

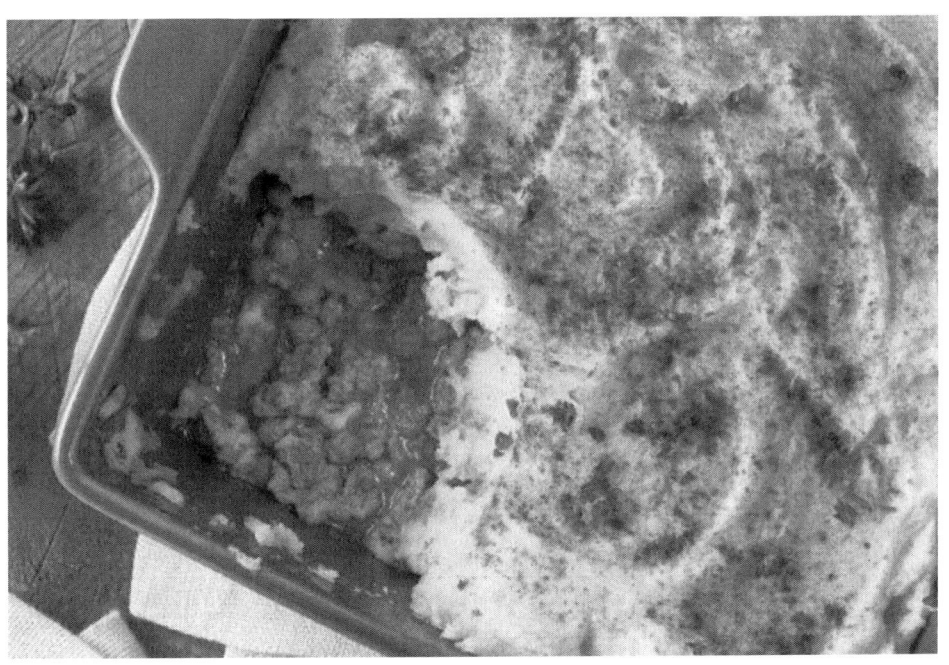

Prep Time:	15 minutes	Calories:	236
Cook Time:	4 hours	Fat (g):	7g
Total Time:	4 hours 15 minutes	Protein (g):	22g
Servings:	6	Net carbs:	23g

Ingredients:

- Chopped onion — ½ cup
- Extra-lean ground beef — 1 pound
- Cornstarch — 1 tbsp
- Water — 1 ¾ cups
- Tomato paste — 2 tbsp
- Chili powder — 1 tbsp
- Worcestershire sauce — 1 tsp
- Frozen mixed vegetables — 1 ½ cups
- Margarine — 2 tbsp
- Garlic powder — ½ tsp
- Potato flakes — 1 1/3 cups
- Milk — 1 cup
- Cheddar cheese, shredded — ¼ cup

Instructions:

1. Cook onions in a large pan with beef for 5 mins.
2. Meanwhile, whisk cornstarch in a half cup of water and add in beef mixture.
3. Put beef in a slow cooker and then add tomato paste, Worcestershire sauce, and chili powder and top with vegetables.

4. In the pan, add 1 ¼ cup water, margarine, and garlic powder and bring to a boil.
5. Add in potato flakes and milk. Spoon over the vegetables and spread evenly.
6. Cover and cook on low for 3-4 hours. Turn off heat and sprinkle cheese.
7. Let stand for 15 mins and serve.

Lo Mein Noodles

"Make these Lo Mein Noodles with some healthy and easy to find ingredients."

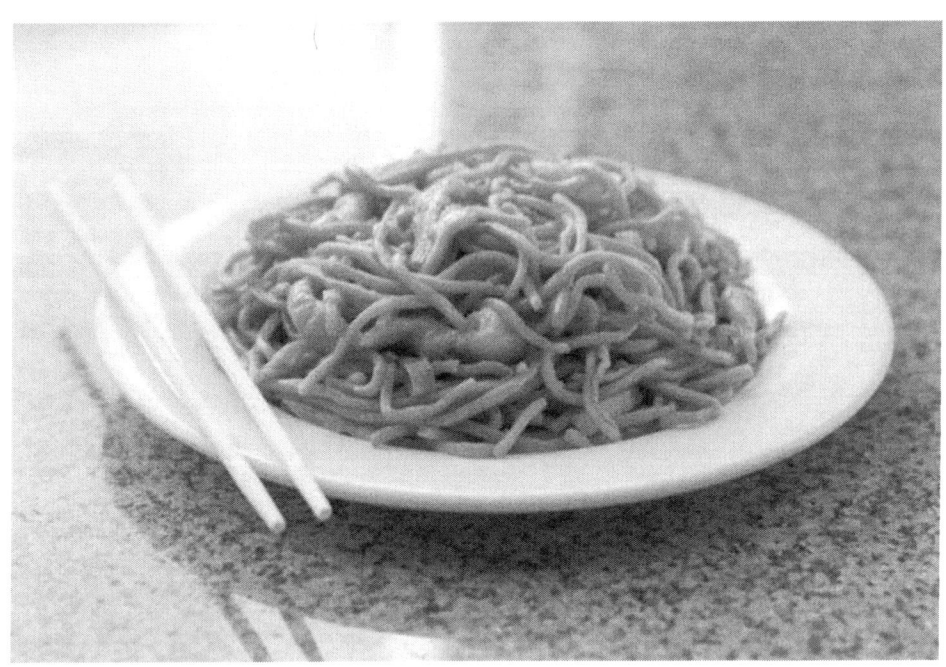

Prep Time:	5 minutes	Calories:	183
Cook Time:	10 minutes	Fat (g):	3g
Total Time:	15 minutes	Protein (g):	7g
Servings:	6	Net carbs:	35g

Ingredients:

- Whole wheat spaghetti — 8 ounces
- Sesame oil — 1 tbsp
- Garlic clove, minced — One
- Carrot, sliced — One
- Snow peas — 1 cup
- Sliced mushrooms — 4 ounces
- Teriyaki sauce — 3 tbsp
- Soy sauce — 2 tbsp
- Honey — 2 tsp
- Grounded ginger — ½ tsp

Instructions:

1. Cook spaghetti as packet instructions.
2. Cook garlic, carrots, and peas with oil in a skillet for 5 mins.
3. Add mushrooms and cook more. In a bowl, mix teriyaki sauce with soy sauce, honey, and ginger.
4. Add the sauce with cooked spaghetti in a skillet and mix.
5. Cook for a couple of mins and serve hot.

Chicken and Dumplings Soup

"Chicken and dumplings are made as a soup in this recipe, and it is a perfect dish for diabetic patients."

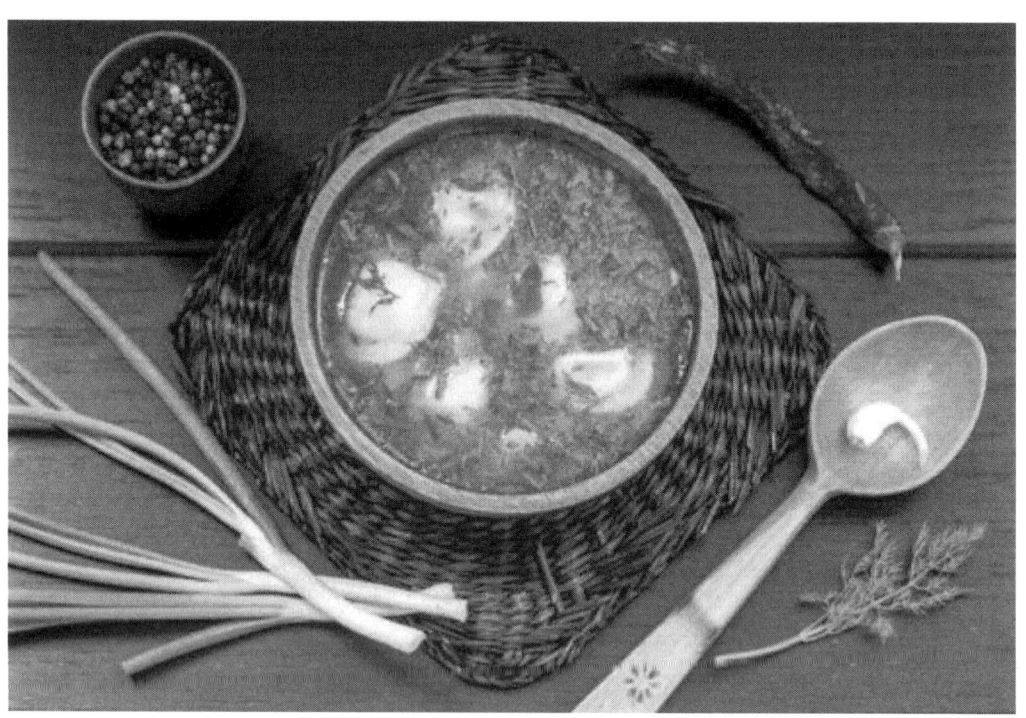

Prep Time:	5 minutes	Calories:	78
Cook Time:	25 minutes	Fat (g):	1g
Total Time:	30 minutes	Protein (g):	11g
Servings:	6	Net carbs:	3g

Ingredients:

- Baking mix   7 tbsp
- Water   3 tbsp
- Dried thyme   ¼ tsp
- Chicken broth   3 ½ cups
- Parsley, chopped   1 tbsp
- Chicken breasts   10 ounces

Instructions:

1. Mix baking mixes with water and thyme and make a soft dough.
2. Boil chicken broth and parsley in a saucepan.
3. Drop the dough using a spoon in the broth. Reduce heat and cook for 10 mins.
4. Add in chicken and cook for 10 mins on low heat.

Sugar-free Pumpkin Bread

"This sweet and spicy pumpkin bread is a real treat for ones who are following a diabetic diet."

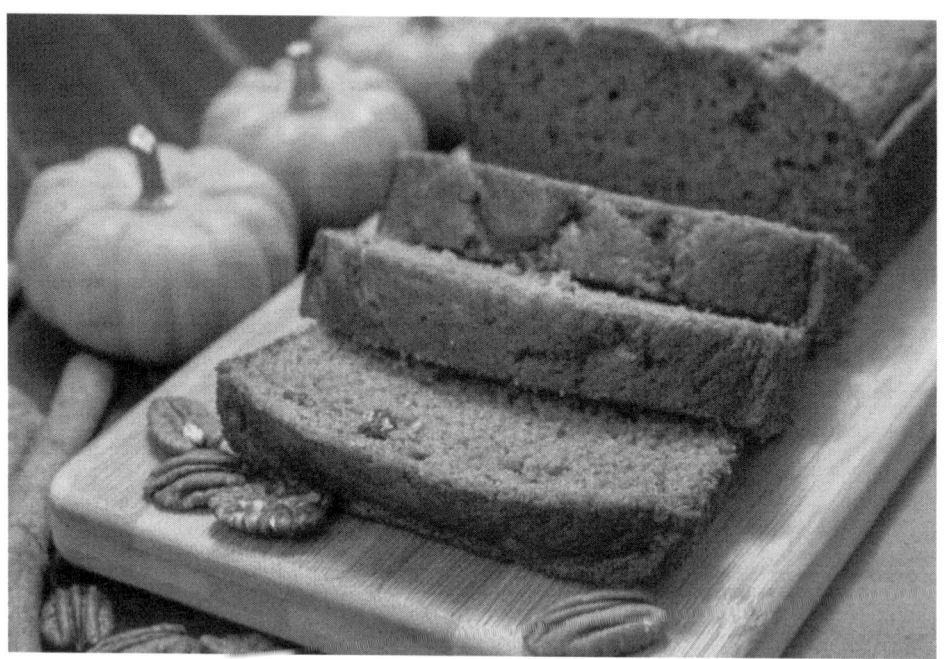

Prep Time:	10 minutes	**Calories:**	66
Cook Time:	55 minutes	**Fat (g):**	2g
Total Time:	65 minutes	**Protein (g):**	2g
Servings:	32 slices	**Net carbs:**	10g

Ingredients:

- Pumpkin — 15 ounces
- Splenda sweetener — 1 cup
- Vegetable oil — ¼ cup
- Low-fat plain yogurt — 1 cup
- All-purpose flour — 1 ½ cup
- Whole wheat flour — 1 ½ cup
- Baking powder — 2 tsp
- Baking soda — 2 tsp
- Cinnamon — 2 tsp
- Salt — ½ tsp
- Raisins — 1 cup

Instructions:

1. Preheat oven to 350 F.
2. In a bowl, mix pumpkin with sweetener, oil, and yogurt and mix well.
3. Take another bowl and add in flours, baking soda, powder, salt, and cinnamon and mix. Then add it in pumpkin mixture and stir well.
4. Add in the raisins and mix.
5. Pour the mixture in a bread loaf pan and bake for 50-60 minutes. Let cool and serve.

Chickpea Flour Tortilla

"This amazing and simple tortilla is made with chickpea flour and is perfectly okay for a diabetic diet."

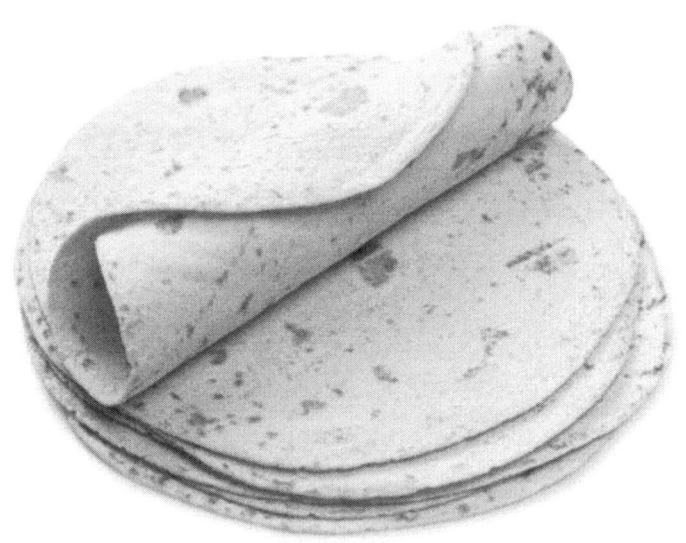

Prep Time:	5 minutes	Calories:	110
Cook Time:	10 minutes	Fat (g):	3g
Total Time:	15 minutes	Protein (g):	5g
Servings:	8 tortillas	Net carbs:	16g

Ingredients:

- Chickpea flour   1 ½ cup
- Bread flour   ½ cup
- Hot water   1 ¾ cup
- Oil   1 tbsp
- Salt   1 tbsp
- Ground black pepper
- Grounded nutmeg   A pinch

Instructions:

1. Take a bowl and combine all of the ingredients and mix to make a consistent batter.
2. Let it rest for a few minutes.
3. In a pan, heat oil and pour the batter and cook until bubbles come up.
4. Flip and cook from the other side too. Serve.

Applesauce Brownies

"These brownies are made with simple and sugar-free ingredients and will satisfy your cravings nicely."

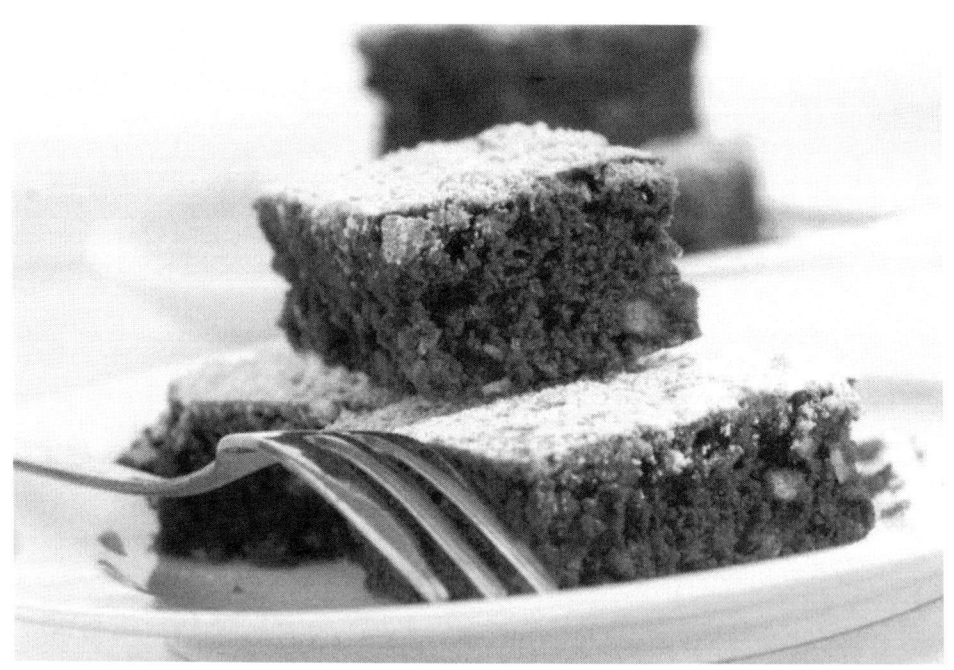

Prep Time:	20 minutes	Calories:	165
Cook Time:	30 minutes	Fat (g):	7g
Total Time:	50 minutes	Protein (g):	3g
Servings:	16	Net carbs:	27g

Ingredients:

- Vegetable oil — 1/3 cup
- Unsweetened applesauce — ½ cup
- Unsweetened cocoa powder — ½ cup
- Sugar, diabetic — ½ cup
- All-purpose flour — 1 cup
- Baking soda — ½ tsp
- Baking powder — 1 tsp
- Eggs — Two
- Vanilla extract — 1 tsp
- Chopped nuts — ¼ cup

Instructions:

1. Preheat oven to 375 F.
2. Mix oil, cocoa, and applesauce and then add in sugar. Mix to dissolve.
3. Add in vanilla and eggs. Mix the dry ingredients and add in the mixture.
4. In a square pan, pour the batter and bake for 25-30 minutes.
5. Cut in squares and serve.

No-Bake Strawberry Cheesecake

"This strawberry cheesecake does not need any baking and is easy and simple to make."

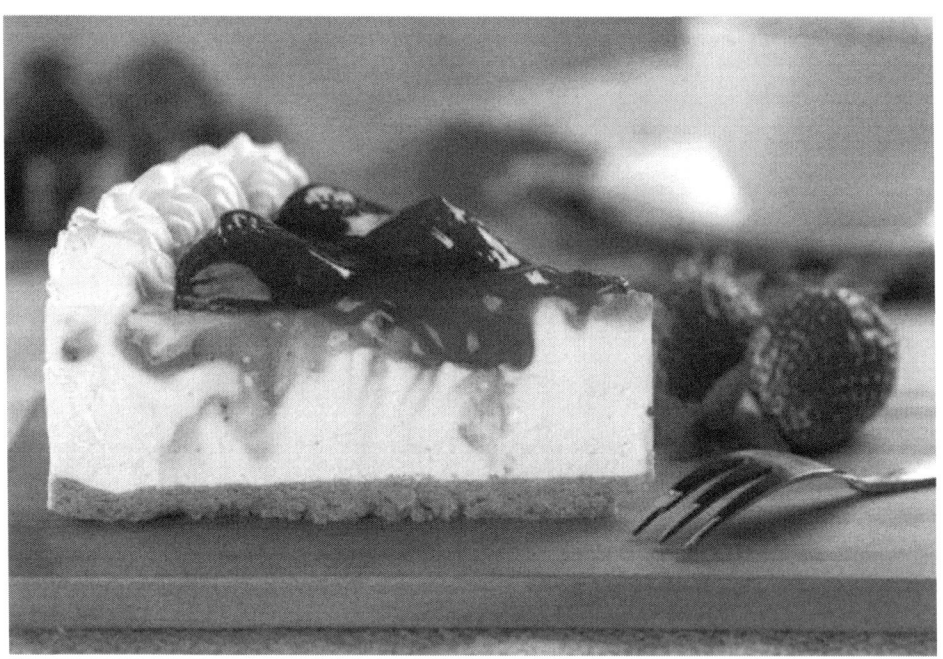

Prep Time:	15 minutes	Calories:	216
Cook Time:	0 minutes	Fat (g):	6g
Total Time:	15 minutes	Protein (g):	5g
Servings:	10	Net carbs:	36g

Ingredients:

- Fat-free cream cheese — 8 ounces
- Sugar substitute — ¼ cup
- Fat-free sour cream — 1 cup
- Vanilla extract — 1 tsp
- Sugar-free frozen whipped topping — 1 ½ cup
- Fresh strawberries, chopped — 1 ½ cup
- Prepared graham cracker pie crust — 9 inch

Instructions:

1. Beat the cream cheese and progressively add sugar and keep beating.
2. Blend in the sour cream and vanilla and then fold the chopped strawberries and whipped topping in it.
3. Place the mixture on the pie crust and keep chill for 4-5 hours.
4. Serve.

Sugar-free Blueberries Coffee Cake

"This coffee cake is stuffed with blueberries and is perfect for those who are following a diabetic diet."

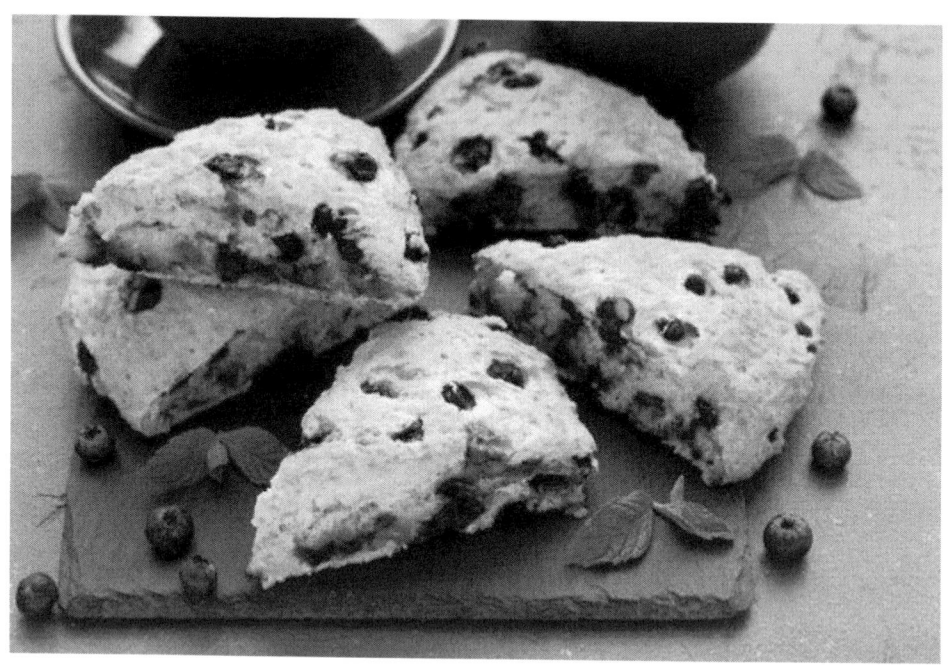

Prep Time:	15 minutes	Calories:	363
Cook Time:	40 minutes	Fat (g):	21g
Total Time:	55 minutes	Protein (g):	6g
Servings:	12	Net carbs:	36g

Ingredients:

- Melted butter — ¾ cup
- Milk — 1 cup
- Eggs — Three
- Vanilla extract — 1 tsp
- Stevia sweetener — 1 ½ cup
- Baking powder — 2 tsp
- All-purpose flour — 3 cups
- Frozen blueberries — 1 ¾ cups
- Brown sugar substitute — 1 ½ cup
- Flour — ¾ cup
- Ground cinnamon — 2 tsp
- Softened butter — ½ cup

Instructions:

1. Preheat oven to 350 F.
2. In a bowl, mix butter, milk, eggs, vanilla, and stevia. Combine the all-purpose flour with baking powder and mix in the wet ingredients.
3. Add in blueberries and spread in a cake pan.
4. In another bowl, mix flour with brown sugar and cinnamon and add in softened butter and mix.
5. Sprinkle over the batter and bake for 40 mins. Serve when done.

Berry Green Smoothie

"Enjoy this simple and easy smoothie recipe with some berries and raw honey."

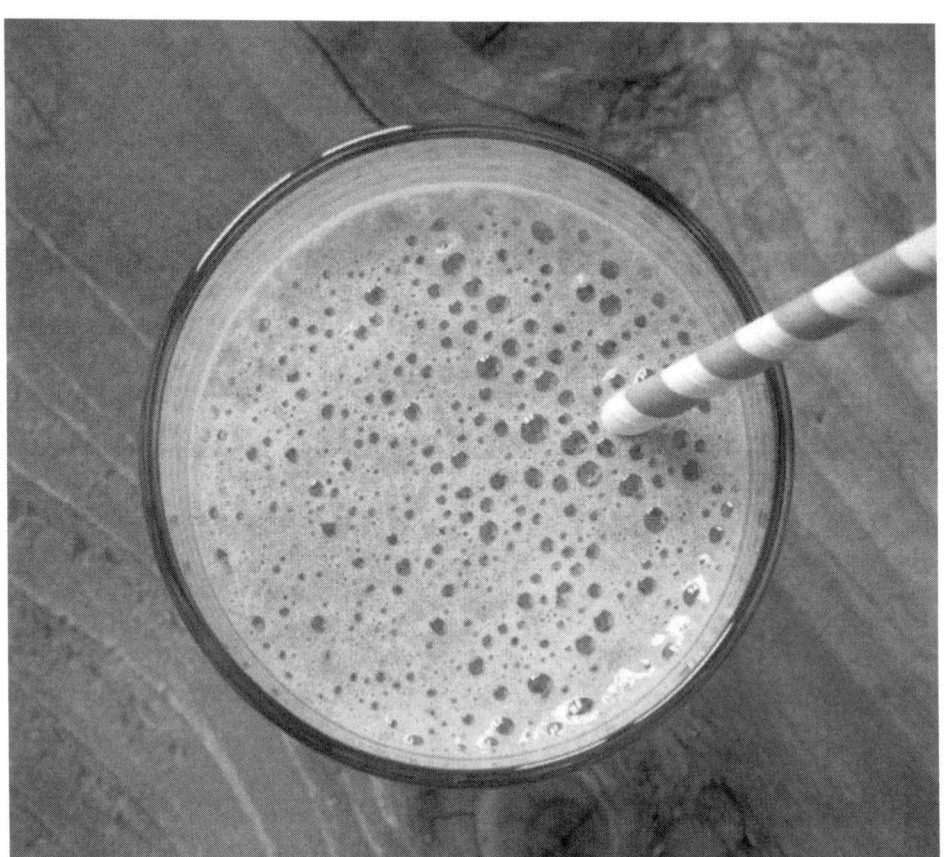

Prep Time:	10 minutes	Calories:	81
Cook Time:	0 minutes	Fat (g):	1g
Total Time:	10 minutes	Protein (g):	2g
Servings:	4	Net carbs:	18g

Ingredients:

- Cranberries — 1 cup
- Raspberries — 1 cup
- Unsweetened almond milk — 1 cup
- Raw honey — 2 tbsp
- Spinach leaves — 3 cups
- Crushed ice — 1 cup

Instructions:

1. Blend all the ingredients in a blender.
2. Keep blending until smooth.
3. Pour in glasses and serve.

Fruits Salad

"Mix up your favorite fruits and do not miss out on a healthy diet."

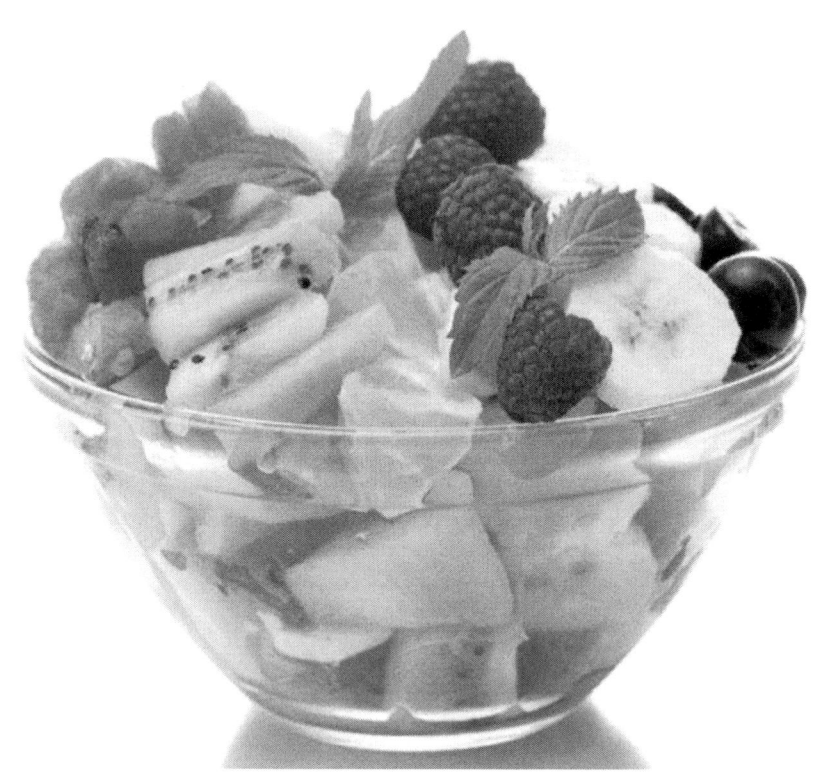

Prep Time:	20 minutes	Calories:	116
Cook Time:	0 minutes	Fat (g):	1g
Total Time:	20 minutes	Protein (g):	1g
Servings:	8	Net carbs:	30g

Ingredients:

- Chopped pineapple — One
- Sliced strawberries — 2 cups
- Lemon, juiced — One
- Cucumber, diced — Half
- Mango, diced — One
- Chilli powder — A pinch

Instructions:

1. Combine pineapple, cucumber, strawberries, and mango.
2. Add in lemon juice and sprinkle chili powder over it.
3. Serve.

Pineapple Salsa

"Enjoy the sweet and sour taste of pineapple, corn, and beans in the form of salsa."

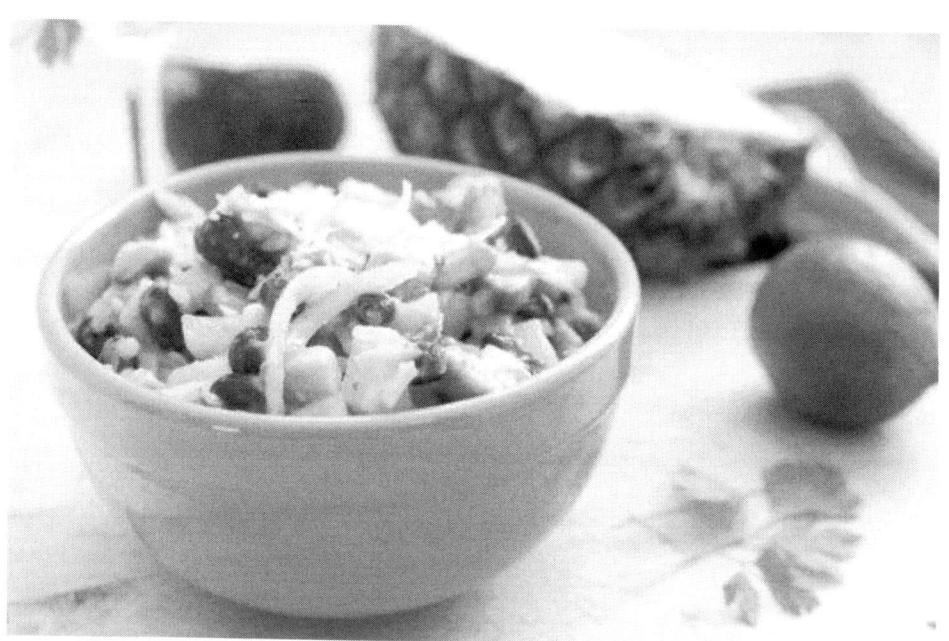

Prep Time:	20 minutes	Calories:	92
Cook Time:	0 minutes	Fat (g):	1g
Total Time:	20 minutes	Protein (g):	4g
Servings:	8	Net carbs:	19g

Ingredients:

- Fresh pineapple, chopped — 1 cup
- Diced red bell pepper — ½ cup
- Diced green bell pepper — ½ cup
- Frozen corn kernels — 1 cup
- Black beans, cooked — 15 ounces
- Chopped onions — ¼ cup
- Chili pepper, green, chopped — Two
- Orange juice — ¼ cup
- Chopped cilantro — ¼ cup
- Ground cumin — ½ tsp
- Salt and pepper — To taste

Instructions:

1. In a large bowl, bring together all ingredients and mix well.
2. Chill and serve.

Strawberries Salad

"Dip the strawberries in sweet and sour dip and enjoy your brunch."

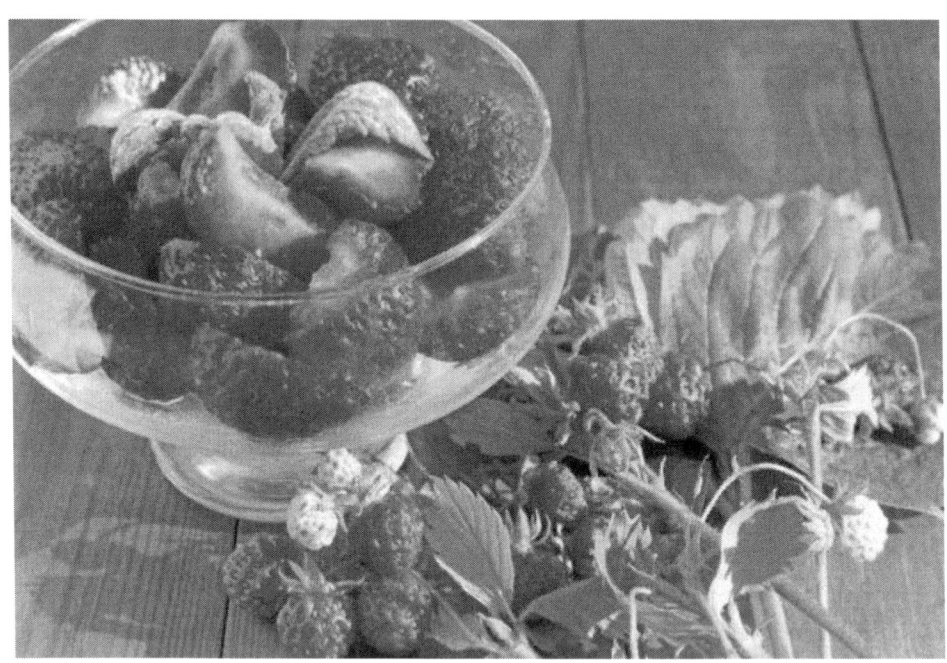

Prep Time:	5 minutes	**Calories:**	89
Cook Time:	0 minutes	**Fat (g):**	1g
Total Time:	5 minutes	**Protein (g):**	1g
Servings:	4	**Net carbs:**	22g

Ingredients:

- Fresh strawberries, sliced   1 ½ pound
- Brown sugar diabetic substitute   2 ½ tbsp
- Balsamic vinegar   1 tbsp
- Grounded black pepper   ¼ tsp

Instructions:

1. In a bowl, combine the strawberries with sugar and let stand for a few mins.
2. In another bowl, mix vinegar with pepper and pour over the berries and mix.
3. Serve.

Creamy Lime Pie

"This simple and easy chilled pie is a perfect diabetic diet option if you are craving a sweet dish."

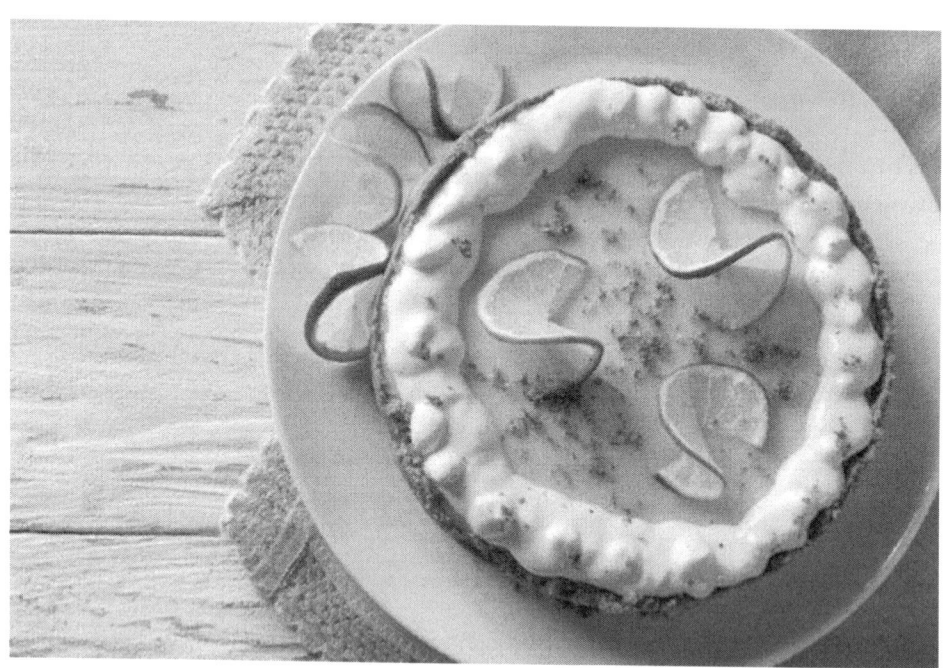

Prep Time:	15 minutes	Calories:	177
Cook Time:	5 minutes	Fat (g):	9g
Total Time:	20 minutes	Protein (g):	2g
Servings:	8	Net carbs:	18g

Ingredients:

- Instant sugar-free lime gelatin mix   4 serving size
- Boiling water   1 cup
- Lime flavored yogurt   2 cups
- Frozen whipped topping   2 cups
- Sugar-free cookie crumb crust   9 inch

Instructions:

1. In a bowl, add gelatin mix in boiling water and mix.
2. Add in yogurt and blend. Add in whipped topping until the mixture is smooth.
3. Spoon the mixture into crust and chill until set. Cut in wedges and serve.

Soda Pop Cake

"This cake is perfect for the ones who are following a healthy and diabetic diet."

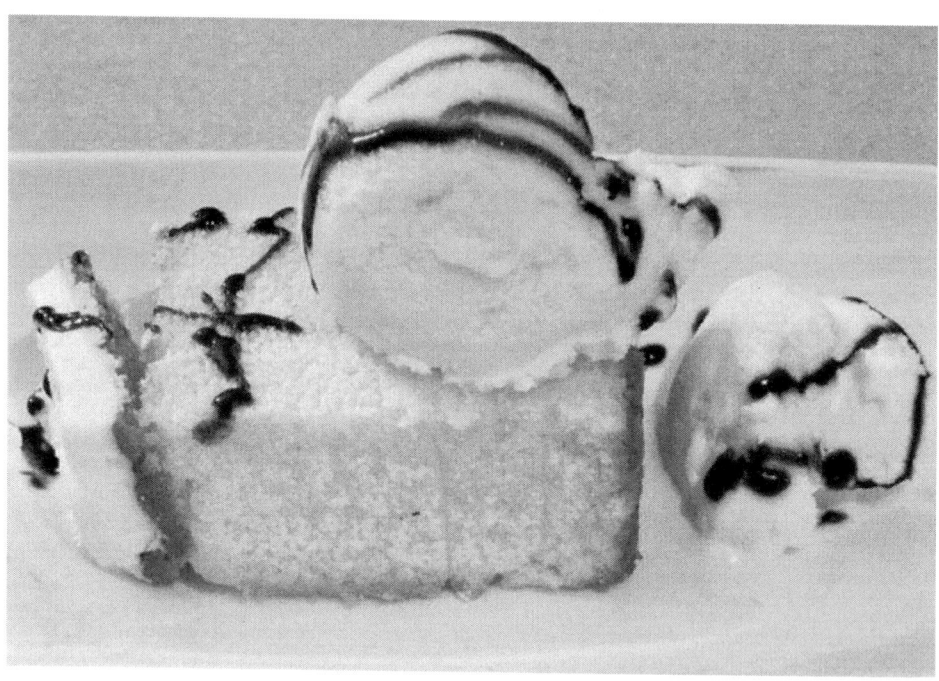

Prep Time:	10 minutes	Calories:	262
Cook Time:	30 minutes	Fat (g):	2g
Total Time:	40 minutes	Protein (g):	1g
Servings:	6	Net carbs:	59g

Ingredients:

- Sugar-free yellow cake mix — 18 ounces
- Diet lemon-lime soda — 12 ounces

<u>Toppings:</u>

- Ice cream topping — 1 ½ cup
- Sugar-free chocolate syrup — ½ cup

Instructions:

1. Preheat oven to 350 F.
2. Add cake mix in a bowl then add in soda and mix.
3. Pour the batter in a cake pan and bake for 25-30 mins.
4. Top with the desired topping and serve.

Caramel Corn Crunch

"Make this sweet and yummy corn crunch for your after evening cravings."

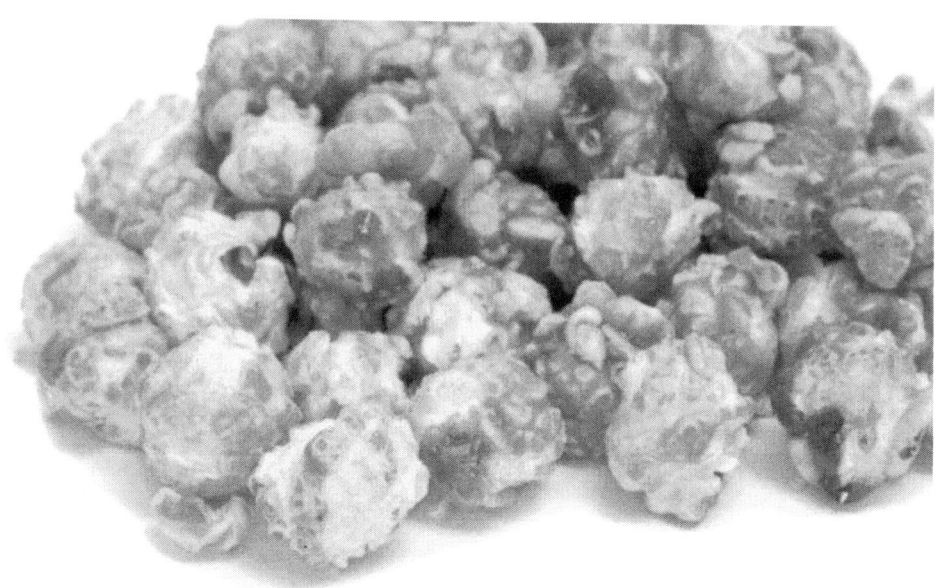

Prep Time:	10 minutes	Calories:	76
Cook Time:	20 minutes	Fat (g):	1g
Total Time:	30 minutes	Protein (g):	1g
Servings:	12	Net carbs:	11g

Ingredients:

- Microwave popcorns — 3 ounces
- Brown sugar substitute — ½ cup
- Margarine — ¼ cup
- Maple flavor syrup substitute — 1/3 cup
- Vanilla extract — 1 tsp
- Baking soda — ¼ tsp

Instructions:

1. Preheat oven to 250 F.
2. Cook popcorns according to the packet instructions. Place in a bowl.
3. In a pan, add sugar, margarine, and maple syrup and cook. Add in vanilla and baking soda and turn off the heat.
4. Pour the syrup on popcorns and spread over the baking sheets.
5. Bake for 20 mins and enjoy.

Sugar-free Cookies

"These simple cookies are sugar-free and have no-calorie sweetener in it, so they are healthy and yummy."

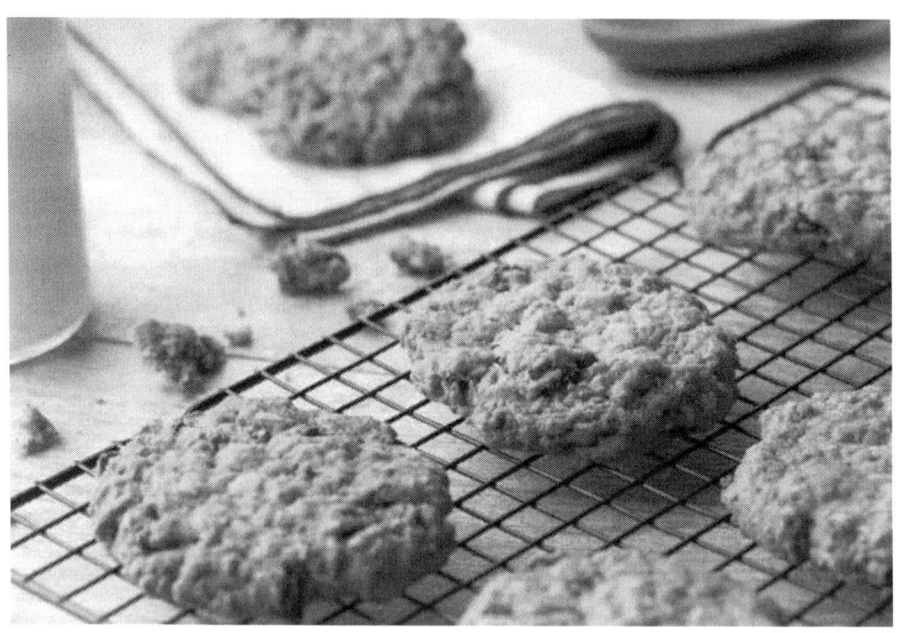

Prep Time:	15 minutes	Calories:	60
Cook Time:	15 minutes	**Fat (g):**	4g
Total Time:	30 minutes	**Protein (g):**	1g
Servings:	48 cookies	**Net carbs:**	7g

Ingredients:

- Unsalted butter — 1 cup
- Splenda sweetener, granulated — 1 cup
- Vanilla — 1 tbsp
- Egg substitute — ¼ cup
- Water — ¼ cup
- Vinegar — ¾ tsp
- All-purpose flour — 1 ½ cups
- Cake flour — 1 ½ cups
- Salt — ¼ tsp
- Baking powder — 1 tsp

Instructions:

1. Preheat oven to 350 F.
2. Beat the butter, sweetener, and vanilla until soft.
3. Add in egg substitute with vinegar and water. Mix well.
4. Add in flour and salt, baking powder, and mix well. Chill dough for 1 hour.
5. Roll out dough on a flat surface and cut with cookies cutter and place on the baking sheet and bake for 13-15 minutes. Let cool and serve.

Sugar-free Frosting

"Do not panic for getting yourself a sugar-free frosting on your cupcakes."

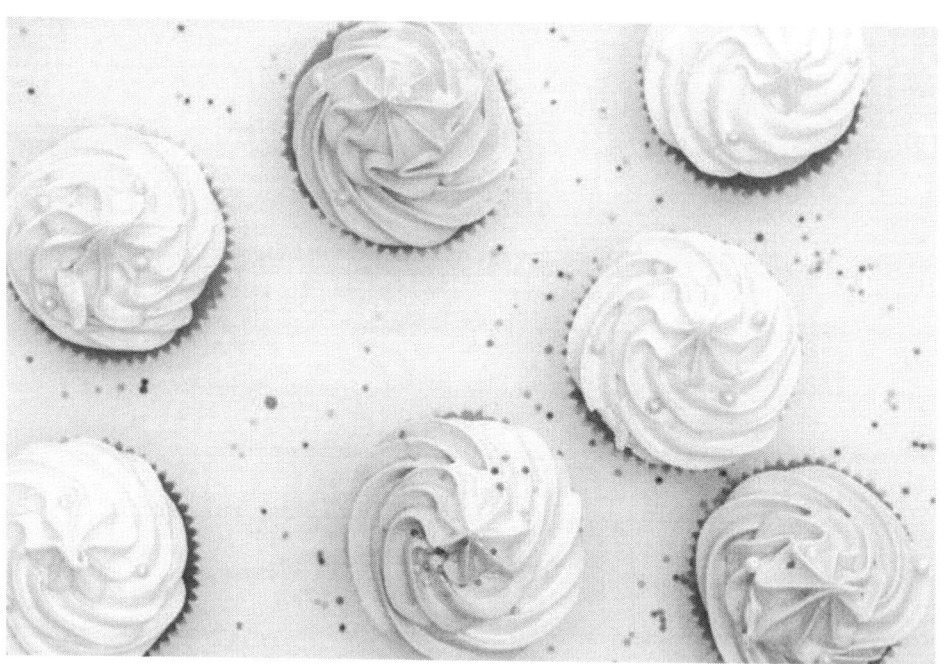

Prep Time:	30 minutes	Calories:	135
Cook Time:	0 minutes	Fat (g):	9g
Total Time:	30 minutes	Protein (g):	2g
Servings:	12	Net carbs:	10g

Ingredients:

- Sugar-free instant pudding mix   1.4 ounces
- Milk   1 ¾ cup
- Cream cheese   8 ounces
- Whipped topping, frozen   8 ounces

Instructions:

1. In a bowl, mix the pudding mix with milk and let sit until thick.
2. Beat cream cheese and add in the pudding.
3. Fold in the whipped topping.

Strawberry and Orange Drink

"This unique and refreshing drink is made with strawberries, orange, and rhubarbs and perfection indeed."

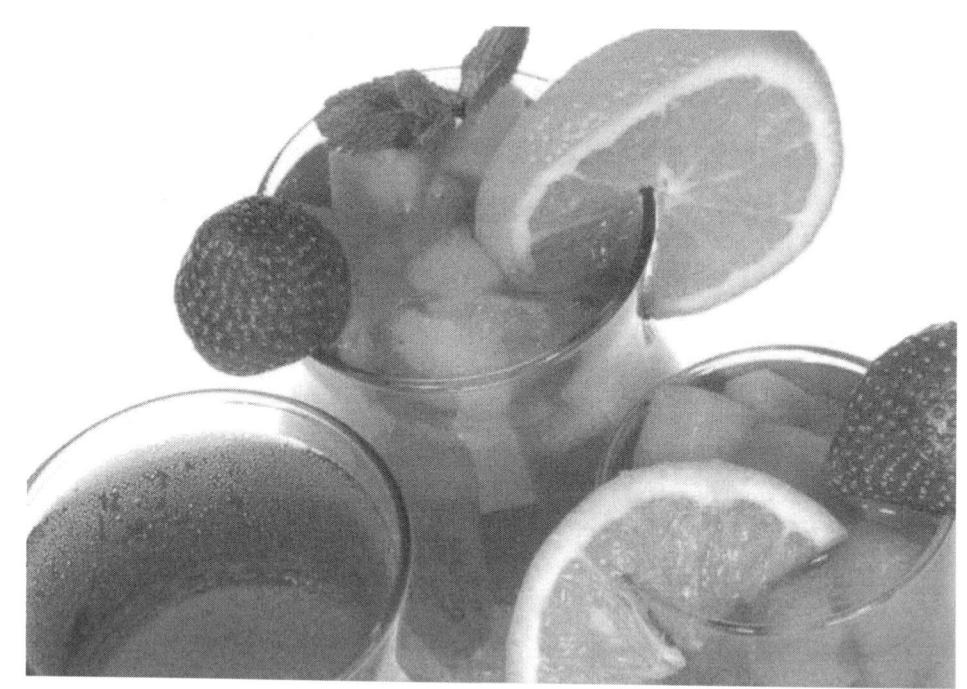

Prep Time:	15 minutes	**Calories:**	30
Cook Time:	25 minutes	**Fat (g):**	0g
Total Time:	40 minutes	**Protein (g):**	0g
Servings:	8	**Net carbs:**	7g

Ingredients:

- Fresh rhubarbs   3 cups
- Coldwater   4 cups
- Sliced strawberries   1 cup
- Orange juice   1 cup
- Mint leaves   For garnish

Instructions:

1. In a large pan, add rhubarb, water and bring to a boil. Simmer for 15 mins more.
2. Let cool for a few minutes and then strain the mixture and drain out the liquid. Discard the pulp.
3. Now pour the liquid in a container and refrigerate for 2 days.
4. For serving, pour the 1/2 cup of refrigerated rhubarb liquid in a jug and add in strawberry slices and muddle to combine well.
5. Add in the remaining liquid along with the orange juice.
6. Garnish and serve.

Sugar-free Pina Colada

"Make this simple and easy Pina colada with sugar-free ingredients."

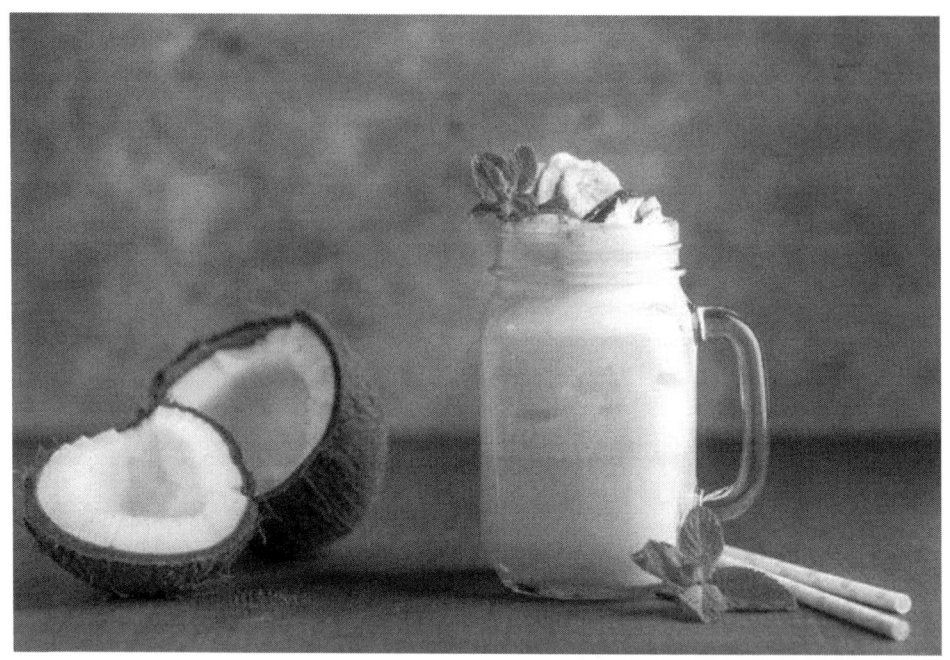

Prep Time:	10 minutes	Calories:	210
Cook Time:	0 minutes	Fat (g):	3g
Total Time:	10 minutes	Protein (g):	1g
Servings:	2	Net carbs:	23g

Ingredients:

- Coldwater — ¼ cup
- Stevia sweetener — 2 packets
- White rum — 3 fl. Oz.
- Lite coconut milk — 1/3 cup
- Ice cubes — A handful
- Frozen pineapple chunks — 12 ounces

Instructions:

1. Add all ingredients in a blender mixer and pulse well. Make a smooth blend.
2. Divide into two glasses and garnish with pineapple slices and serve.

Spinach and Artichoke Dip

"Try this amazing and yummy dip made with artichoke and spinach. It is a perfectly healthy and simple food to enjoy."

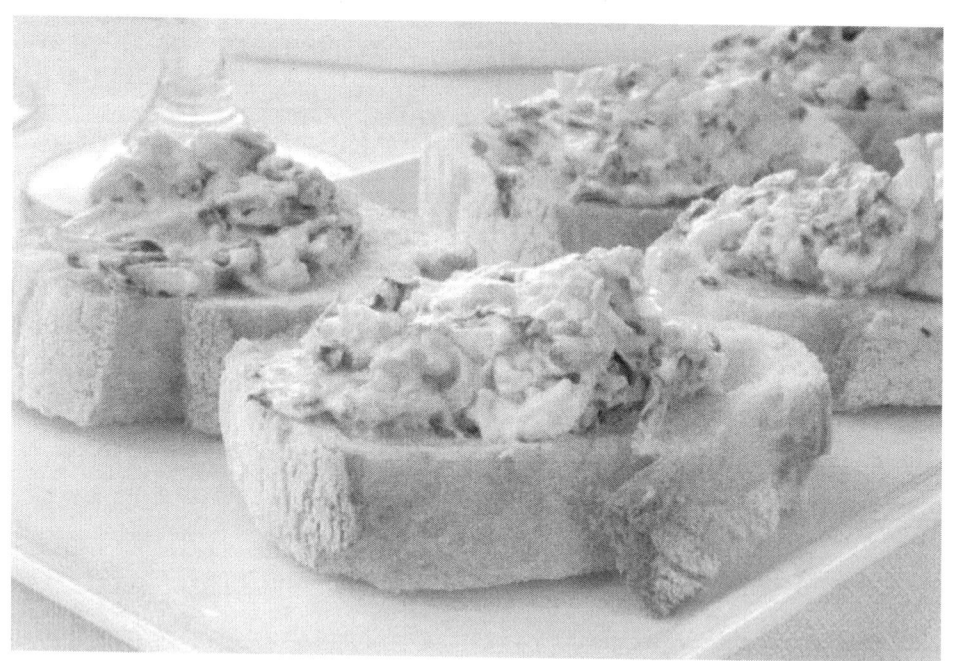

Prep Time:	10 minutes	Calories:	179
Cook Time:	25 minutes	Fat (g):	12g
Total Time:	35 minutes	Protein (g):	11g
Servings:	8	Net carbs:	7g

Ingredients:

- Artichoke hearts, chopped — 14 ounces
- Frozen spinach, chopped — 10 ounces
- Low-fat yogurt — 8 ounces
- Shredded mozzarella cheese — 1 cup
- Green onion, chopped — ¼ cup
- Garlic clove, minced — One
- Chopped red pepper — 2 tbsp

Instructions:

1. Preheat oven to 350 F.
2. Combine all ingredients except the red pepper and mix well.
3. Pour it in a casserole dish and bake for 22-25 mins.
4. Sprinkle with red pepper and serve.

Springtime Dip

"This easy dip is made with yogurt and buttermilk and is healthy for eating with any snacks."

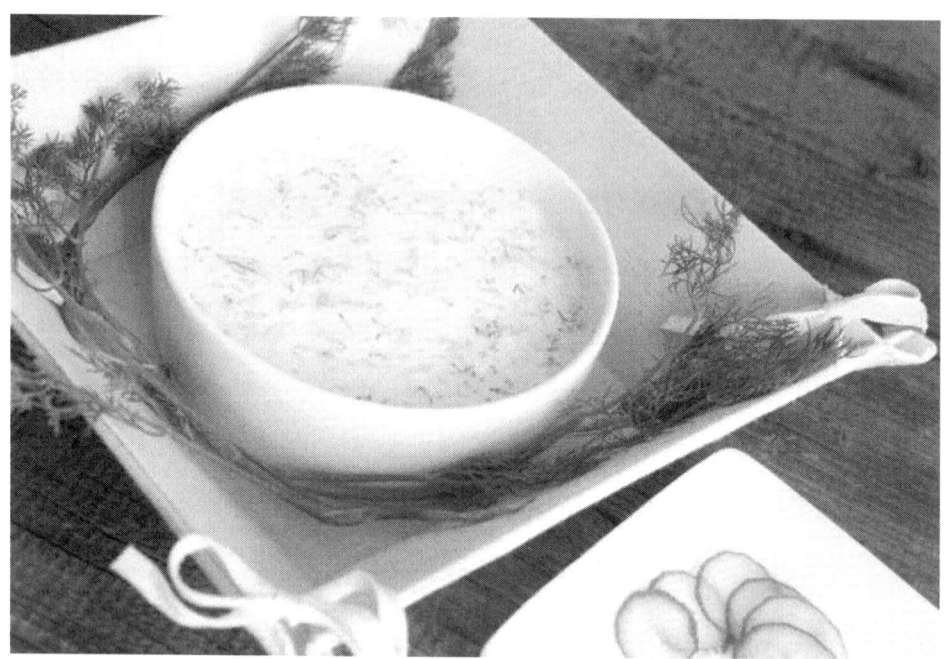

Prep Time:	5 minutes	Calories:	33
Cook Time:	0 minutes	Fat (g):	0.2g
Total Time:	5 minutes	Protein (g):	5g
Servings:	6	Net carbs:	3g

Ingredients:

- Fat-free Greek yogurt — 1 cup
- Buttermilk — ½ cup
- Lemon juice — 1 tsp
- Chopped fresh dill — 1 tbsp
- Garlic powder — ½ tsp
- Black pepper — ¼ tsp
- Lemon peel — ½ tsp

Instructions:

1. Take a small bowl and add all ingredients one by one.
2. Whisk to well combine.
3. Serve after chill.

Spicy Red Sauce

"Make this delicious red sauce which is spicy and sweet at the same time and is easy to make."

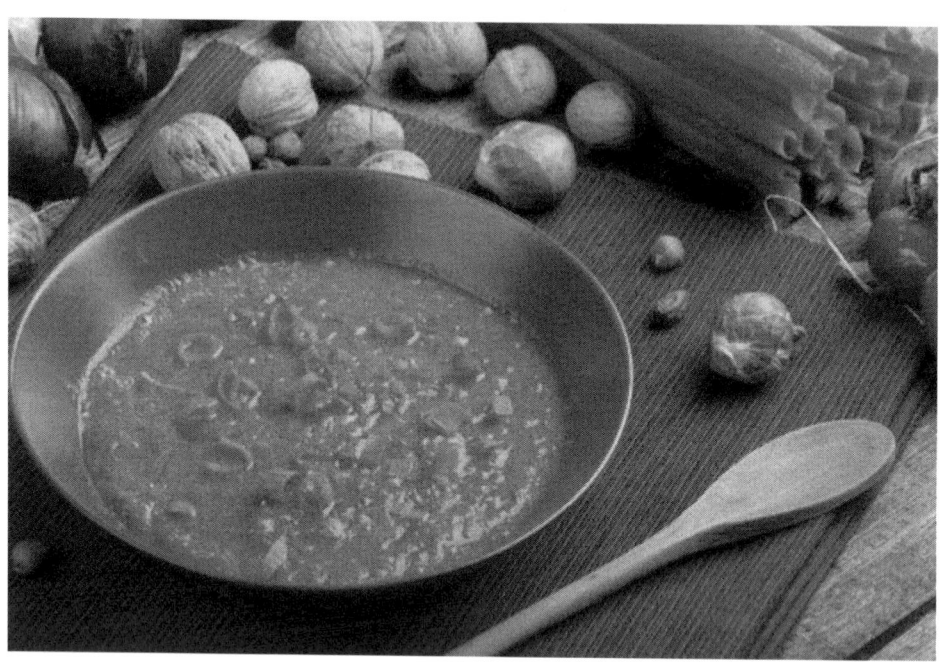

Prep Time:	5 minutes	Calories:	72
Cook Time:	15 minutes	Fat (g):	1g
Total Time:	20 minutes	Protein (g):	2g
Servings:	6	Net carbs:	16g

Ingredients:

- Frozen tricolor pepper and onion blend — 14 ounces
- Minced garlic cloves — Three
- Crushed tomatoes — 28 ounces
- Water — ½ cup
- Italian seasoning — 1 tsp
- Crushed red pepper — ½ tsp
- Splenda — 2 tsp

Instructions:

1. Cook vegetables and garlic on medium heat in a saucepan.
2. Add in crushed tomatoes once vegetables are tender, followed by water, Splenda, and red pepper and bring to a boil.
3. Reduce heat and cook for 12-15 mins.

Printed in Poland
by Amazon Fulfillment
Poland Sp. z o.o., Wrocław